# ATLAS OF
# FACIAL NERVE SURGERY

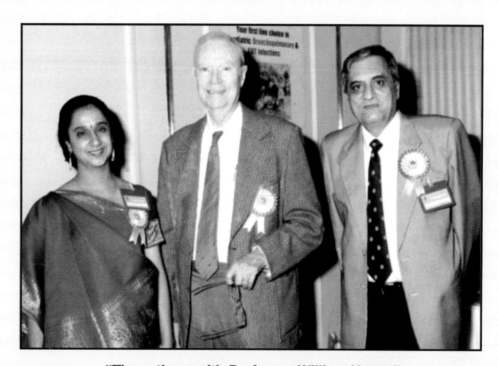

*"The authors with Professor William House"*

# ATLAS OF FACIAL NERVE SURGERY

**DS Grewal**

MS DORL FACS

Professor and Head of the Department

President, Association of Otolaryngologists of India (AOI) – 2005-06

Vice Chairman–Indian Academy of Otolaryngology

**Bachi T Hathiram**

MS DORL DNB

Associate Professor

President AOI, Mumbai – 2003-04

Hon. Associate Secretary AOI – 2005-06

Department of ENT and Head and Neck Surgery

TN Medical College and BYL Nair Ch. Hospital

Mumbai, India

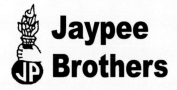

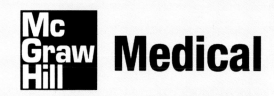

ISBN     0-07-148576-7
ISBN 13  9780071485760

# List of Contributors

**Anesthesia for Otologic Surgery**
**CM Deshpande**
Associate Professor
Dept. of Anesthesiology
TN Medical College and BYL Nair Ch. Hospital
Mumbai, India

*and*

**AN Modi**
Lecturer
Dept. of Anesthesiology
TN Medical College and BYL Nair Ch. Hospital
Mumbai, India

**All Sketches by**
**Mohammed Hashmi**
Senior Registrar
Dept. of ENT and Head & Neck Surgery
TN Medical College & BYL Nair Ch. Hospital
Mumbai, India

**Facio-hypoglossal Jump Anastomoses for Reanimation of the Paralyzed face**
**J J Manni**
Head of the Department
Otorhinolaryngology and Head and Neck Surgery
University Hospital, Maastricht
The Netherlands

**Tumors Causing Facial Palsy**
**David Moffat**
Consultant Surgeon and Chairman
Dept. of Otoneurological and Skull Base Surgery
Addenbrooke's Cambridge University Hospital
Cambridge, UK

**Testing of Facial Nerve**
**Alok Mohorikar**
Chief Resident
Dept. of ENT and Head and Neck Surgery
TN Medical College and BLY Nair Ch. Hospital
Mumbai, India

*and*

**Vicky Khattar**
Senior Resident
Dept. of ENT and Head and Neck Surgery
TN Medical College and BYL Nair Ch. Hospital
Mumbai, India

**Surgery of the Paralyzed Face**
**Narendra Pandya**
Diplomate, American Board of Plastic Surgery
Hon. Cosmetic Surgeon
Jaslok Hospital
Breach Candy Hospital
Ex Hon. Prof. of Plastic Surgery
TN Medical College and BYL Nair Ch. Hospital
Mumbai, India

*and*

**Ashok Shah**
Hon. Asst. Professor, Grant Medical College and
The Sir J.J. Group of Hospitals,
Consultant Plastic Surgeon
Harkisondas Hospital
Breach Candy Hospital
Mumbai, India

# Foreword

It gives me immense pleasure to write a foreword for this Atlas, as I know the authors Dr DS Grewal and Dr Bachi T Hathiram personally. This Atlas has brought up many thoughts about my experience with the surgical management of the facial nerve.

I finished my residency in ENT at the County Hospital in Los Angeles in July 1956. I joined my brother Howard in his busy practice that was mostly otology. A few months later we imported the first Zeiss surgical microscope in the US. To me it provided a wonderful new look at the temporal bone and opened many new surgical possibilities.

At that time many radical mastoids were done for chronic infection and cholesteatoma to open up the mastoid spaces for drainage. Cure of the infection was not an option. Granulation often covered the middle ear and surrounded the facial nerve. I had been taught that if the facial nerve was so much as touched, it was thought a weakness or paralysis would occur. For this reason the granulation was left to continue draining, but at least the infection would not break into the brain.

The microscope, however allowed gentle elevation of the granulation and careful observation of the facial nerve in its the middle ear portion. I learned amazingly, that touching the facial nerve did not cause facial weakness.

Gradually, that rather than staying away from the facial nerve, I began to identify and use it as a landmark to orient to the structures of the middle ear and mastoid. This led to thoughts that if Bell's palsy was due to swelling of the nerve in the bony canal, maybe removing bone over the middle ear and mastoid part of the nerve would relieve the pressure on the nerve. The technique of the microscope combined with continuous suction irrigation and diamond stone bone removal, was developed. The results were not spectacular but sometimes the weakness of the face would improve right after surgery.

At the same time I had begun to develop the middle fossa approach to the internal auditory canal. The problem was to open the internal auditory canal from above without damaging the facial nerve. I found that by identifying the greater superficial petrosal nerve, following it back to the geniculate ganglion, and then uncovering the nerve as it led down to the internal auditory canal, that I could see everything I needed to see. Again the facial nerve was a friendly landmark rather that a feared no man's land.

This book reviews the many aspects of facial nerve pathology and surgery. There are more than 200 intra-operative photographs—the result of their vast experience over several decades of surgery. This Atlas also incorporates the work of several other experienced surgeons in the field. Otologists today must have this knowledge if they are to serve the best interests of their patients. I hope you, the reader, can be inspired to take this knowledge, learn it well, and then extend it further, for the benefit of mankind.

**William F House** DDS MD
President, AllHear, Inc.

# Preface

The Facial Nerve has fascinated and interested almost all Otologists since several decades leading to extensive studies being carried out on the nerve and it's functions. Inspite of this, a comprehensive atlas featuring various intraoperative photographs of the facial nerve and its pathologies is conspicuous by its absence.

My fascination with the facial nerve goes back several decades when I operated more and more cases of carcinoma of the cheek. Earlier, the trend was to functionally reconstruct the face postoperatively and this was achieved by reconstructing the outer and inner lining of the cheek. However, invariably, this was followed by sagging of the face. According to my experience, there was a failure to realize that, with the inner and outer lining of the cheek there is a middle layer, which includes the facial nerve and hence, is most important from the functional and cosmetic viewpoint. This concept got me interested in facial nerve surgery, and slowly and steadily prompted me to study facial nerve in the middle ear.

The conception of the "Atlas" however was not only because of my keen interest in the facial nerve but also in the art of photography for which I received professional training from the Indo-American Society, Bombay in 1976. The magic of photography is that it allows you to capture a moment before it is gone. I personally believe that a photograph should be such that once the audience sees it, they should be able to visualize the mind of the photographer, and actually feel the pulse of the subject. Pondering over a photograph later may also help a surgeon to observe something new that was previously unnoticed and give him ideas to improvise on his technique.

In my experience, the facial nerve can be considered as the most photogenic structure in the middle ear due to its long and tortuous course. It is best captured on a photograph as it does not reflect light but absorbs it. Its exact intraoperative color is best seen in the light of the operating microscope, photographed without the use of a flash. All these features of facial nerve along with a good surgical exposure make the facial nerve an interesting subject for an atlas. The constant use of Zeiss operating microscopes have significantly contributed to the quality and precision of my photography.

Also, I would like to emphasize that the facial nerve should be considered very much as a part of mainstream ENT surgical practice and should be dealt with confidence by trainee and budding otologists, rather than being scared of it and avoiding it. The purpose of this atlas is to achieve this through exhaustive photographic depiction of the nerve and it's various features (anatomical and pathological), which will allow the young otologist to visualize and indeed understand this so called complex structure as a thing of beauty, and fall in love with the facial nerve. Surgery of facial nerve has proven to increase the chance of cure and hence the perspective towards surgical treatment needs to be changed.

I would like to thank our **Dean, Dr Sanjay Oak** and our **ex-Dean Dr G V Koppikar** for giving me all the facilities for facial nerve surgery. I would also like to thank *Dr L H Hiranandani,* my constant source of inspiration as well as *Dr N L Hiranandani* my colleague and friend; **Prof William House**, a legend in Otoneurosurgery for writing the foreword; **Prof John Ballantyne** one of our senior colleagues and a renowned otologist who has always guided me; *Dr David Moffat, Cambridge; Dr Johannes J Manni, Netherlands; and Dr Narendra Pandya, Dr Ashok Shah, Dr CM Deshpande, and Dr AN Modi, India;* for their contribution. I am thankful to *Dr Mohammed Hashmi* for drawing the diagrams for the Atlas. I also would like to thank my lecturer, *Dr Nilam Sathe* and my past and present residents – Dr Manoj Bhaskaran, Dr Trupti Manjrekar, Dr Neha Shah, Dr Paresh Tankwal, Dr Rahul Mehta, Dr Ashwin Dwivedi, Dr Shobhit

Srivastava, Dr Ritu Agarwal, Dr Lovneesh Kumar, Dr Santhosh Davis, Dr Minal Shroff, Dr Rajeev T, Dr Mukesh Kumar, Dr Vijay Prakash, Dr Palak Shroff, Dr Prashant Sharma and Dr Mitul Chamadia, as they were associated during various stages of preparation of the Atlas. *My special thanks to Dr Alok Mohorikar and Dr Vicky Khattar who have not only contributed a chapter, but have worked tirelessly with us throughout the making of this Atlas. Dr Sonal Saraiya* was a great help in the proofreading of the Atlas. I would also like to thank **Dr Rohan Walvekar** and **Dr Kaushal Sheth**, my past residents for all their help in the basic stages of the Atlas.

I sincerely hope that this Atlas serves its purpose of enlightening the readers about the various aspects of the facial nerve and the photographs capture the essence of facial nerve surgery, which is important for maintaining the normalcy of the face – truly the index of man.

The facial nerve is considered as a "friend of the otologist" and through our experience, we feel that the facial nerve sheath is a boon to the otologist as it is not only a barrier in limiting the spread of disease to the facial nerve but, also prevents iatrogenic trauma to the nerve. This firm belief of mine forms the principle of unhesitant atraumatic facial nerve surgery.

I am indeed grateful to my colleague and co-author of this atlas, **Dr Bachi T Hathiram** for making this belief a reality.

Jointly through this Atlas, we have made an effort to familiarize you with our concepts of facial nerve surgery.

**Dr DS Grewal**

# Contents

**DVD includes**

"Operative video clippings-
The Otologist's perspective"

# CHAPTER 1
# Anatomy of the Facial Nerve

The facial nerve is the nerve of the second branchial arch. It is a mixed nerve. The course of the seventh cranial nerve can be broadly classified into (Fig. 1.1):
  i. Intracranial
  ii. Intratemporal
  iii. Extratemporal.

## SUPRANUCLEAR PATHWAY

The facial nucleus is represented in the precentral gyrus of the cerebral cortex. The facial nerve fibres run downwards from the precentral gyrus through the genu of the internal capsule and then through the pons where majority of the fibres cross over to reach the opposite facial nerve nucleus. Some fibres continue on the same side to terminate in the ipsilateral nucleus.

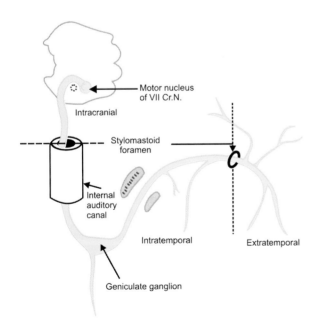

**Figure 1.1**

Diagrammatic representation of the course of the facial nerve

The facial nerve nucleus is located in the pons ventrolateral to the abducens nucleus. The fibres of the facial nerve emerging from the facial nucleus curve around the abducens nucleus and later pass ventrolaterally and downwards to lie between the facial nucleus and the spinal nucleus of the trigeminal nerve. They emerge from the lower border of the pons between the olive and the restiform body as a motor root and a sensory root (nerve of Wrisberg) and it is from here that the infranuclear pathway starts.

## INFRANUCLEAR PATHWAY

The facial nerve after leaving its nucleus travels along with the eighth cranial nerve in the cerebellopontine angle to enter the internal auditory canal (IAC). The facial nerve consists of a motor root, carrying fibres to the muscles of the second pharyngeal arch (muscles of facial expression, scalp, auricle, stylohyoid, stapedieus and the posterior belly of the digastric). While the sensory root consists of:
- Special visceral afferent: taste to anterior 2/3rd of the tongue via the chorda tympani.
- General visceral efferent: salivary glands via the petrosal nerves.
- Special visceral efferent: to the facial muscles.

Upon entering the porus (IAC), the seventh cranial nerve and the nervus intermedius join to form a common trunk, which lies slightly above and anterior to the eighth cranial nerve. A dural prolongation containing a narrow subarachnoid space and spinal fluids surrounds the seventh and the eighth cranial nerves to the lateral end of the internal auditory canal (fundus) (Fig. 1.2). After leaving the internal auditory canal, the facial nerve enters a separate bony canal, the fallopian canal (Fig. 1.3) in the temporal bone.

The facial nerve has a unique course through the long, narrow and tortuous bony fallopian canal in its

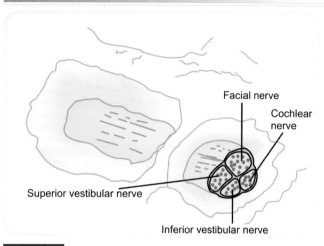

**Figure 1.2**

Diagrammatic representation of course of facial nerve through the internal auditory canal

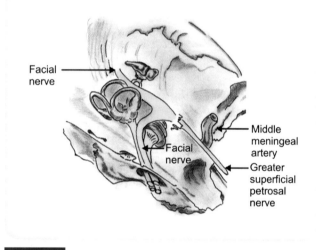

**Figure 1.3**

Diagrammatic representation of labyrinthine and tympanic segment of the facial nerve

intratemporal segment. This renders it more susceptible to damage following trauma or disease pathology and the symptoms depend on which portion of the nerve is involved.

The total length of the facial nerve in the temporal bone is 22-33 mm, and its course can be broadly subdivided into the following segments:

1. The first horizontal segment from the fundus of the internal acoustic meatus to the geniculate ganglion is 3-5 mm in length and is known as the labyrinthine segment.

2. The nerve then takes an acute angled turn to enter the tympanic cavity. This is the first genu.
3. It then runs posteriorly on the medial wall of the middle ear above the promontory forwards to backwards. This is the tympanic segment and is 10-12 mm in length.
4. It then curves down at the pyramid and oval window at an angle. This is the second genu.
5. The mastoid segment or the vertical segment runs from the second genu to the stylomastoid foramen and is 9-16 mm in length.

As the nerve enters the facial (fallopian) canal 3 morphologic peculiarities are noted as described by Gerrier (1977):

a. Individual sheath of pia mater curves up and continues with arachnoid.
b. Slight constriction of nerve is seen just prior to its labyrinthine segment about 0.68 mm (Fisch U,1981) in diameter, which is a normal constriction of the nerve.
c. Change in the direction of the nerve that produces an angle of 132 degrees, open anteriorly and medially.

## Labyrinthine Segment

Contains the seventh nerve and nerve of Wrisberg, inclined slightly from above to below and from behind to forwards. It is 3-5 mm in length and extends from the fundus of the internal acoustic meatus to the geniculate ganglion.

First turn of the facial nerve and the geniculate fossa: The geniculate fossa is the crossroad of four-nerve canals, i.e.

• Central and peripheral extremities of the facial canal.
• Conduit for the greater superficial petrosal nerve.
• Conduit for the lesser superficial petrosal nerve.

The fossa is quadrangular in shape measuring 2-3 mm. It is completely enclosed in a bone, but it is occasionally only covered with dura. The geniculate fossa contains the geniculate ganglion—the bulbous enlargement of the facial canal. The nerve of Wrisberg terminates in the ganglion but emerges as the greater superficial petrosal nerve passing through the facial hiatus.

## Second Part or Tympanic Segment (Fig. 1.3)

The facial canal is horizontal and 10-12 mm in length. It extends from the geniculate fossa to the posterior wall of the tympanum. It is inclined slightly inferiorly and forms an angle of less than 10 degrees with the plane of the horizontal canal. It does not give any branches in this segment.

## Second Turn of the Facial Canal or Second Genu

It is a curvature with a wide radius which starts in the horizontal plane and then becomes almost vertical. The angle formed varies from 95 to 125 degrees.

## Vertical/mastoid Segment

It extends from the second genu to the stylomastoid foramen measuring 9 to 16 mm in length. It forms an angle of 95 to 125 degrees with the tympanic portion of the facial canal (second genu). It runs through the mastoid process. The vertical portion tends to swing laterally and at the level of the stylomastoid foramen the nerve is found more superficial than at the level of the second genu.

The second genu lies beneath the posterior portion of the horizontal semicircular canal. The facial canal is separate from the posterior fossa by a distance of 4-5 mm; this retrofacial space is usually occupied by retrofacial air cells. The mastoid portion of the facial canal deviates posteriorly from the vertical by 5-35 degrees.

We have observed that in the mastoid portion just prior to entering the stylomastoid foramen, the nerve takes a distinct obtuse angled turn forward towards the foramen deviating from its vertical course. This is an important landmark for the stylomastoid foramen. We term this as the *third genu* (Figs 1.4 a and b).

## Stylomastoid Foramen

Opens at the base of the petrosa between the mastoid and styloid groove facing forward towards the base of the styloid process. In the newborn, the stylomastoid foramen is at a higher level with the facial nerve emerging at the level of the mastoid antrum.

## Extratemporal Facial Nerve

After it emerges from the stylomastoid foramen the nerve turns anteriorly in the substance of the parotid gland, and divides at the posterior border of the ramus of the mandible into two primary branches.

Superior (temporofacial) branch which is larger and horizontally directed.

Inferior (cervicofacial) branch which is smaller and longer and vertically directed.

From this, a plexiform arrangement of nerves arises called the parotid plexus or the Pes Anserinus (as it resembles goose feet), which are distributed over the head, face and upper part of the neck. In the parotid gland the facial nerve presents a curvilinear course and then as it emerges from the parotid it rapidly becomes superficial and is related to the external wall of the parotid space which is a thin glandular bed.

## Branches of the Facial Nerve (Fig. 1.5)

### Intracranial

Greater superficial petrosal nerve: It is the first branch, which arises from the geniculate ganglion and carries secretomotor fibres to the lacrimal gland.

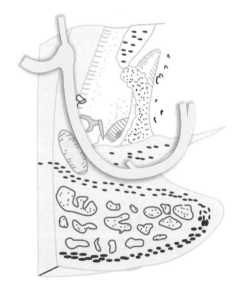

**Figure 1.4 a**

Diagrammatic representation showing the angulation of the facial nerve anteriorly prior to entering the stylomastoid foramen (third genu)

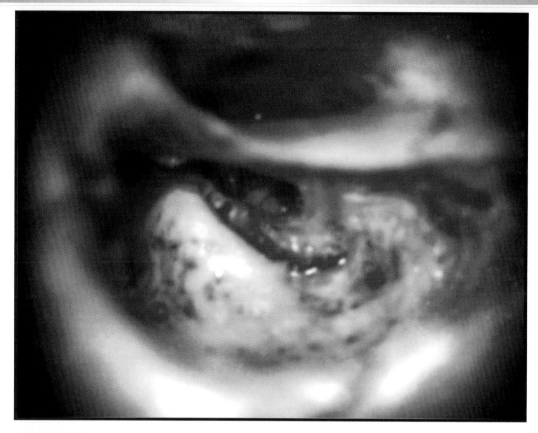

**Figure 1.4 b**

Intraoperative photograph showing the third genu

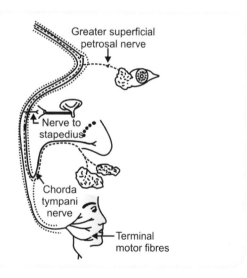

**Figure 1.5**

Diagrammatic representation of the branches of the facial nerve for topodiagnostic tests

*Greater superficial petrosal nerve*

*Nerve to stapedius*

*Chorda tympani nerve*

*Terminal motor fibres*

**Intratemporal branches:** which arise from the mastoid segment:

1. *Nerve to the stapedius muscle*—arises from the mastoid segment and supplies the stapedius muscle.

2. *Chorda tympani nerve*— arises from the mastoid segment, slightly more distal to the nerve to the stapedius, courses anteriorly across the middle ear space between the incus and malleus to join the lingual nerve and supplies the anterior 2/3rd of the tongue. It also supplies secretomotor fibres to the submandibular gland.

3. The *sensory fibres* of the nerve which join the auricular branch of the vagus and supply the skin of the external auditory canal.

### Branches of Facial Nerve in the Neck and Face

1. The Ansa Haller (inconstant) which arises immediately below the stylomastoid foramen and anastomoses with the glossopharyngeal nerve while passing lateral to the jugular vein.
2. Posterior auricular branch arises 1 to 2 mm below the stylomastoid foramen, winds around the digastric muscle and extends posteriorly upon the anterior surface of the mastoid. There it is joined by a filament from the auricular branch of the vagus and communicates with the posterior branches of the greater auricular nerve and with the lesser occipital nerve. Between the external auditory canal and the mastoid process it divides into auricular and occipital.
3. Stylohyoid branch frequently arises in conjunction with the digastric branch and enters the stylohyoid muscle in its mid portion.
4. Branch to the posterior belly of digastric muscle.
5. The lingual branch, which follows the styloglossus muscle and replaces the Ansa Haller.

### Branches that form the Parotid Plexus

1. Temporal branches of facial expression.
2. Zygomatic branches of facial expression.
3. Buccal branches of facial expression.
4. Marginal mandibular branch, which supplies orbicularis oris and muscles of lips and chin.
5. Cervical branch which supplies the platysma.

### Surgical Landmarks of the Facial Nerve

Anatomical landmarks provide the surgeon with various ways to locate the facial nerve, which is distorted by trauma, tumour or infection.

### Landmarks for Extratemporal Part

The pinna is important since the incision for all facial nerve surgeries is decided on its position. Parotidectomy is the most common procedure in which the extra-temporal facial nerve is dissected. Different methods to locate the nerve during surgery are:

   i. Tragal pointer (of Conley)—The nerve is located medial and about 1 cm inferior to the tragal cartilage.
  ii. Tympanomastoid suture—This is located at the apex of the vagino-mastoid angle or valley of the nerve. It is the angle where the vaginal process of the tympanic portion of the temporal bone meets the mastoid process. The facial nerve runs just deep to this suture.
 iii. Styloid process—The nerve passes lateral to the styloid process at the skull base.
  iv. By tracing the terminal branches of the facial nerve backwards:
   • The ramus frontalis is located by a line from the tragus to lateral canthus.
   • The ramus buccalis is located by a line from the tragus towards the alae of the nose parallel to the zygoma but 1 cm below.
   • Ramus mandibularis is near the angle of the mandible at a point 4-4.5 cm from the attachment of the lobule of the pinna.
   v. Tendon of the posterior belly of digastric muscle.
  vi. Posterior auricular vein or the Retromandibular vein.

During submandibular gland excision, to save the marginal mandibular branch, dissection should be carried out in the plane deep to the fascia overlying the submandibular gland.

### Landmarks in the Mastoid and the Middle Ear

   i. The cog, which is a bony ridge, which hangs from the tegmen, anterior to the head of the malleus, is useful in identifying the first genu.
  ii. Cochleariform process is immediately inferior to the anterior portion of the tympanic segment of the facial nerve. When the cochleariform process is inapparent it may be located by identifying the Jacobson's nerve on the promontory and tracing it superiorly.
 iii. The oval window is a useful guide to the posterior portion of the horizontal segment of the nerve. The nerve lies above the oval window.
  iv. The lateral semicircular canal lies posterosuperior to the second genu. This is a very constant landmark.
   v. Retrofacial air cells help in delineating the medial aspect of the vertical segment of the facial nerve.

5

vi. The chorda tympani is used as a landmark when performing a Combined Approach Tympanoplasty.

vii. The upper portion of the vertical segment lies in the base of the bony ridge that separates the sinus tympani from the facial recess. The processus pyramidalis attaches to the superior aspect of this ridge.

viii. Digastric ridge points to the lateral and inferior aspect of the vertical segment of the facial nerve.

ix. The nerve is located medial to the inferior portion of the tympanic annulus.

x. In our experience, while decompressing the facial nerve in case of trauma and palsy due to injury/tumour/disease, most of these anatomical landmarks are destroyed but we have observed a constant relation of the facial nerve in the angle formed by the posterior canal wall and the floor of the mastoid. The posterior canal wall meets the floor of the mastoid below the lateral semi-circular canal with an inclination and forms an angle with it. The facial nerve lies within the apex of this angle. (Fig. 1.6) Using a 2-3 mm diamond burr to drill the mastoid bone the facial nerve can be easily exposed in this angle. By further thinning the posterior meatal wall anteriorly the facial recess is opened.

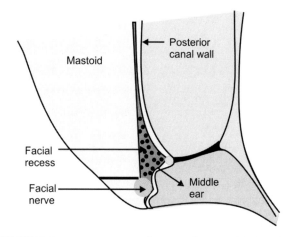

**Figure 1.6**

Diagrammatic representation of the relation of facial nerve to the posterior canal wall and floor of the mastoid

## Landmarks in the Middle Cranial Fossa

The Middle cranial fossa approach being a neuro-surgical approach, most of the otologists are not familiar with it. The standard landmarks are different from the ones used in the mastoid, middle ear and the parotid. These include the greater superficial petrosal nerve, which is the most common landmark. The greater superficial petrosal nerve is identified and followed backwards to the geniculate ganglion and the facial nerve is identified. Another landmark is the identification of the internal auditory canal. The external auditory canal and the internal auditory canal lie in the same coronal plane. Drilling is begun in the same plane as the external auditory canal and then the internal auditory canal is identified followed subsequently by the geniculate ganglion and the facial nerve. Also, the bulge of the superior semicircular canal can be identified and subsequently the internal auditory canal is identified.

## Anatomical Variations and Anomalies Involving the Facial Nerve and its Canal

All components of the temporal bone are subject to variation—The facial canal may display:
   a. Congenital bony dehiscence.
   b. Variations and anomalies of its usual course.
   c. Rarely, a persisting embryonic artery or vein may also be seen.

## Congenital Bony Dehiscence

A gap in the continuity of the bony fallopian canal may be observed in any portion. It is more commonly seen in the tympanic portion (Fig. 1.7) and it may involve the medial, inferior or lateral walls. Most frequent site is above and posterior to the oval window. Occasionally the dehiscence may be near the cochleariform process or over the superior aspect and medial to the geniculate ganglion. Occasionally, there may be more than one site of dehiscence. Baxter (1971) has derived more accurate information concerning the site and incidence of dehiscence from histological examination of temporal bones at Massachusetts Eye and Ear Infirmary. In a series of 535 temporal bones, dehiscence was detected in 55%

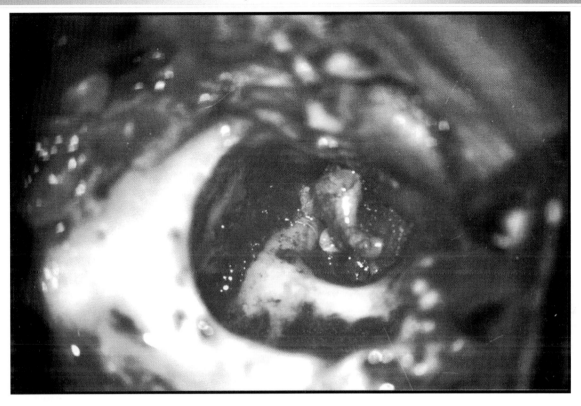

**Figure 1.7**

Intraoperative photograph showing a dehiscence of the bony    fallopian canal in the tympanic segment

cases out of which 91% were intratympanic and 9% were in the mastoid segment. Of all the dehiscences in the tympanic segment, 83% were located adjacent to the oval window (Figs 1.8 a and b) involving the lateral, medial and inferior portion with the facial nerve protruding from its bony canal in 26%. In less than 1% the dehiscence involved the entire tympanic segment.

### Variation of the Course of the Facial Nerve

Fowler (1961) collected the most pertinent forms of literature and his observations were as follows:
- Variations involving the mastoid segment may be found in a normally developing temporal bone.
- A variation involving the tympanic segment frequently is associated with a lack of differentiation or agenesis of the oval window.
- Severe dysplasias of the middle ear or inner ear are regularly accompanied by an aberrant course of the nerve.

Aberrant course of the nerve is classified according to the site at which it occurs:
a. *Canalicular segment (Intracranial segment)*—The canalicular segment may enter the petrous pyramid instead of going through the internal acoustic meatus, through the subarcuate fossa and may run through the center of the superior semicircular canal to the stylomastoid foramen bypassing the middle ear cavity as described by Dworacek (1960). Bifurcation of the nerve may be seen.
b. *Labyrinthine segment*—Bifurcation of the labyrinthine segment may be seen rarely as described by Altmann (1933) and Miehlke and Partsch (1963).
c. *Tympanic segment*—
   1. Facial nerve crossing along the superior aspect of the lateral semicircular canal has been documented by House as described by Nager and Proctor (1991).

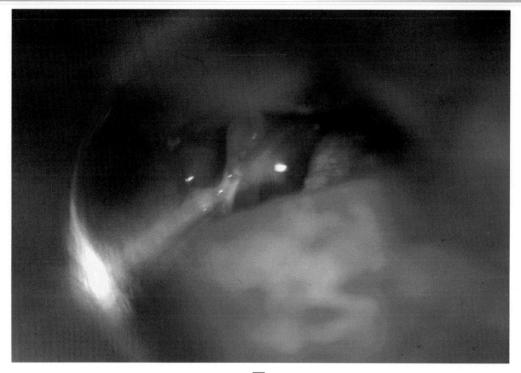

a

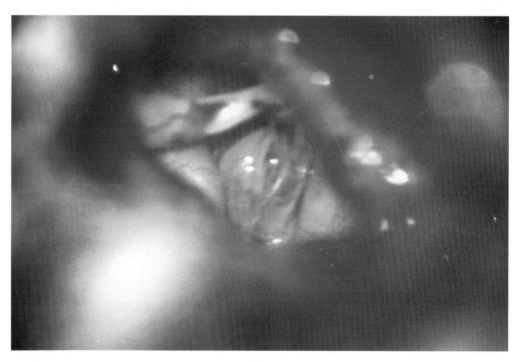

b

**Figures 1.8 a and b**

Intraoperative photograph showing facial nerve overhang

2. Bifurcation of the nerve anterior or proximal to the oval window has been noticed by Nager and Proctor (1991), Baxter (1971), Dietzel (1961) and Fowler (1961) (Fig. 1.9).
3. Facial nerve crossing horizontally over the oval window (Figs 1.10 a and b).
4. Facial nerve crossing through the stapedial arch as documented by Butler (1968), Caparosa and Kalassen (1966) and Ombre-danne (1960).
5. Nerve crossing posteriorly between the oval and round windows as described by Durcan et al (1967) (Fig. 1.11).
6. Facial nerve crossing postero-inferiorly to the round window.
7. Facial nerve passing from the geniculate ganglion straight downwards over the promontory anterior to both oval and round windows and exiting through the hypotympanum as reported by Dickinson et al (1968) (Fig. 1.12).
8. Hypoplasia of the facial nerve as seen by Kodama et al (1982).

d. *Anomalies of the mastoid segment*—
1. Most frequent is a posterior and lateral bulge (dorsal hump) of the canal beneath the prominence of the lateral semicircular canal as described by Fowler (1961) and Kettel (1946) (Fig. 1.13).
2. The nerve may follow an abnormal posterior, lateral or anterior course as seen by Kettel (1963) (Fig. 1.14).
3. Bifurcation of the facial nerve posterior or distal to the oval window with the two branches continuing in separate canals and the mastoid process through separate foraminae has been

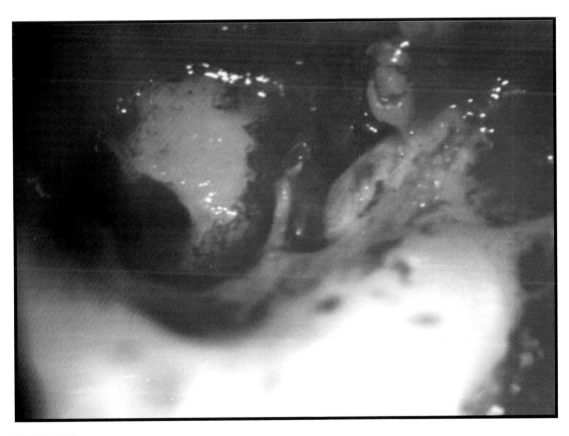

**Figure 1.9**

Intraoperative photograph of a bifid facial nerve in the tympanic segment (proximal to the oval window)

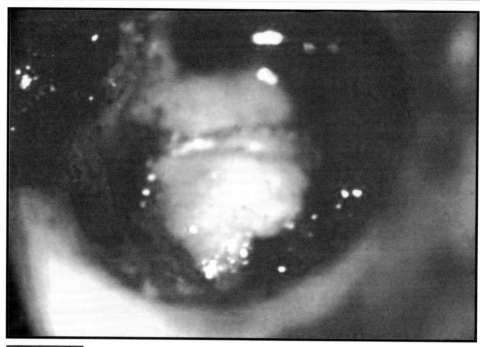

**Figure 1.10 a**

Intraoperative photograph of tympanomastoidectomy showing the seventh nerve running over the stapes footplate

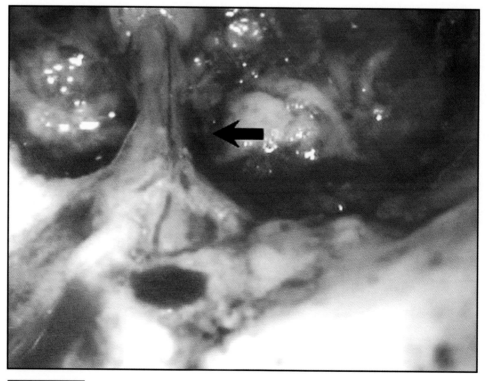

**Figure 1.10 b**

Intraoperative photograph showing the facial nerve running over the stapes footplate with only the small inferior portion of the footplate being seen (arrow)

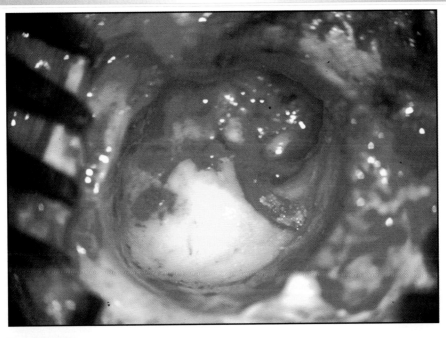

**Figure 1.11**

Intraoperative photograph of the anomalous facial nerve which is anteriorly displaced and running between the round window and the stapes footplate over the promontory

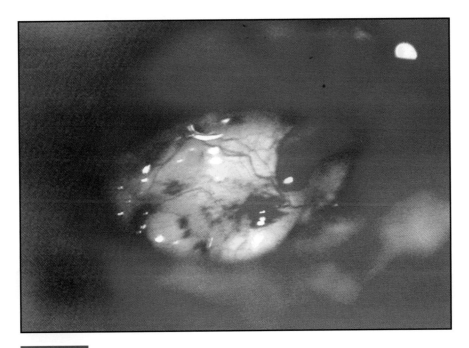

**Figure 1.12**

Intraoperative photograph of exploratory tympanotomy showing facial nerve running over the promontory. The round window is covered by bone

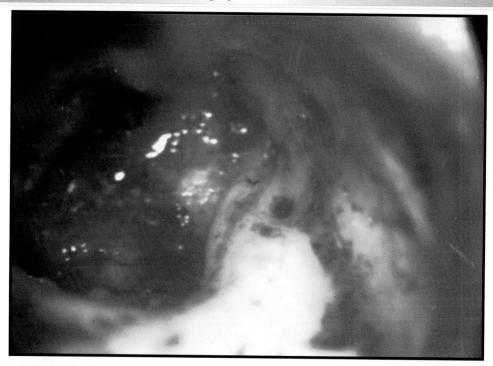

**Figure 1.13**

Tympanomastoid surgery showing an anteriorly placed facial nerve in relation to the lateral semicircular canal

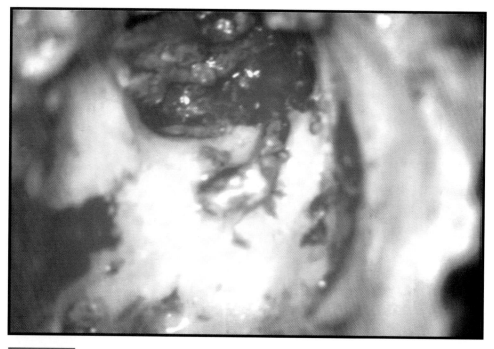

**Figure 1.14**

Intraoperative photograph of a dehiscent facial nerve entering the middle ear through aditus ad antrum and running posterior to its normal course in the mastoid segment mentioned by Arndt (1967), Hahlbrock (1960) and Mielhke (1973). The separate branches may join on their way into a single trunk before passing through the stylomastoid foramen or just outside it as seen by Arndt (1967) and Wright (1981) (Figs 1.15 and 1.16). Occasionally, the nerve is trifurcated.

4. Hypoplasia of the nerve.
5. Anomalous branches arising in the mastoid segment (Fig. 1.17).

### Anatomic Variation in the Extratemporal Course of the Facial Nerve

Though the facial nerve terminates into its terminal branches within the parotid gland the branching pattern is extremely variable. Various researchers have studied this. However, the most recent study is by Katz and Catalano (1987) where they have classified this branching pattern into 5 types:

*Type I (25%)*
  a. splitting and reunion of the zygomatic branch
  b. splitting and reunion of the mandibular branch

*Type II (14%)* Buccal branch fuses distally with the zygomatic branch

*Type III (44%)* Major communication between the buccal branch and the other branches

Type IV (14%) complex anastomotic branching patterns between the major divisions

Type V (3%) Facial nerve leaves the skull as more than 1 trunk.

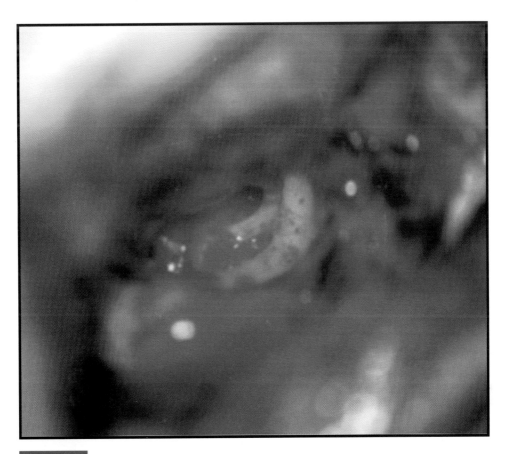

**Figure 1.15**

Exploratory tympanotomy showing a bifid facial nerve over the promontory

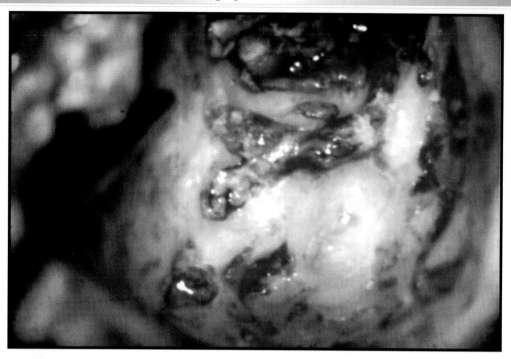

**Figure 1.16**

Tympanomastoid surgery showing a bifid facial nerve in the mastoid segment

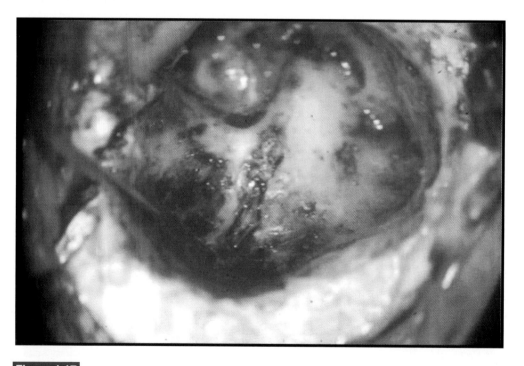

**Figure 1.17**

Intraoperative photograph of tympanomastoid surgery showing a branch of facial nerve to the occipitofrontalis muscle abnormally arising from the mastoid segment and running across the mastoid cavity

## Anatomic Variations of Chorda Tympani

The origin varies from 1 mm distal to 11 mm proximal to the stylomastoid foramen as described by Nager and Proctor (1991). Rarely, bifurcation may occur as reported by Durcan et al (1967).

## Abnormal Veins and Arteries along the Facial Nerve

A persistent stapedial artery may be encountered in the tympanic segment of the facial nerve through the stapedial arch. In a rare instance, a large vein of equal size or larger than the nerve may be observed joining the nerve in the facial canal near the geniculate ganglion, accompanying it to the stylomastoid foramen. The vein represents a persistent lateral capital vein.

## Facial Nerve Sheath

Throughout the fallopian canal, the nerve (and its two infrageniculate branches) is enclosed in a fibrous sheath. As exposed during surgical procedures this sheath consists from without inwards of:

1. A tough, shiny, grey periosteal layer.
2. A vascular plane of arteries and venous plexus embedded in loose connective tissue.
3. A firm fibrous layer perforated by the vessels and on its deep surface in contact with the perineural connective tissue.

Although a clear plane of dissection is found between the sheath and the nerve, this plane is crossed by innumerable connective tissue strands, which require careful division and separation if a length of the nerve is to be decompressed.

At the internal auditory meatus the sheath blends with the dural coverings of the nerve, while at the stylomastoid foramen it fuses with the periosteum and with the adjacent facial layers covering the diagastric muscle, the parotid gland and carotid vessels. The sheath is easily recognized under the operating microscope and it is a valuable barrier against mechanical injury and infection. It should be incised only if there are proper surgical indications for doing so.

## Blood Supply of the Facial Nerve

Within the confined space of the fallopian canal special attention to the blood supply of the nerve is necessary. A detailed account is given by Blunt (1954). The stylomastoid artery, a branch of the occipital artery, enters the stylomastoid foramen and runs upwards anterior and slightly medial to the nerve, sending short branches at intervals around and into it. At the geniculate ganglion the petrosal branch of the middle meningeal artery enters the canal and runs distally to anastomose with the stylomastoid artery. Within the internal auditory meatus the nerve is supplied by the internal auditory artery and in the posterior cranial fossa by the anterior inferior cerebellar artery. The veins form a plexus around the nerve, from which efferent vessels run obliquely, first between the sheath and the nerve and then through the sheath to lie on its outer surface. Apart from small veins accompanying the chorda tympani, the venous drainage leaves the canal mainly at the stylomastoid foramen and at the second genu.

The anterior inferior cerebellar artery, petrosal branch of middle meningeal artery and stylomastoid branch of posterior auricular artery anastomose proximal to the geniculate ganglion. Facial nerve is vulnerable to ischemia in the labyrinthine segment. Sympathetic nervous control of vasomotor tonus is presumed to be effective through the cervical sympathetic fibres distributed around the branches of the external carotid artery.

## BIBLIOGRAPHY

1. Altmann F: "Zur anatomie und formalen genese der atresia auris Congenita". Monatasschr Ohrenheilkd Laryngorhino 1933;67:765-71.
2. Arndt HJ: "Zweiteilung des nervus facialis zwischen ganglion geniculi und foramen stylomastoideum"; HNO (Berlin) 1967;15:116-18.
3. Baxter A: "Dehiscence of the fallopian canal": Journal of Laryngology and Otology 1971;85:587-94.
4. Butler GE: "Transtapedial congenital malposition of the facial nerve"; Archives of Otolaryngology 1968;88:268.
5. Caparosa RJ, Klassen D: "Congenital anomalies of the stapes and facial nerve"; Archives of Otolaryngology 1966;83:420-21.

6. Dickinson JT, Srisomboon P, Kamerer DB: "Congenital anomaly of the facial nerve"; Archives of otolaryngology 1968;88:357-59.

7. Dietzel K: "Ueber die Dehiszenzen des Facialis Kanals"; Z Laryngology Rhinology Otology 1961;40:366-76.

8. Durcan DJ, Shea JJ, Sleeckx JP: "Bifurcation of the Facial nerve"; Archives of Otolaryngology 1967;86:619-31.

9. Dworacek H: "Die anatomischen Verhaltnisse des Mittelohres unter operations microscopischer Betrachtung"; Acta Otolaryngologica (Stockholm) 1961;51:31-45.

10. Fisch U: "Surgery for Bell's palsy"; Archives of Otolaryngology 1981;107:1-11.

11. Fowler EP Jr: "Variations in the temporal bone course of the facial nerve"; Laryngoscope 1961;71:937-44.

12. Gerrier Y: "Surgical anatomy particularly vascular supply of the facial nerve". In Fisch U (Ed): Facial Nerve Surgery. Birmingham, AL, Aesculapius, 1977.

13. Hahlbrock KH: "Zweiteilung des N facialis im warzenfortsatz"; Arch Ohren Nasen Kehlkopfheilkd 1960;174:465-70.

14. Katz AD, Catalano P: "The clinical significance of the various anastomotic branches of the facial nerve. Report of 100 patients"; Archives of Otolaryngology Head Neck Surgery 1987;113(9):959-62.

15. Kettel K: "Abnormal course of the facial nerve in the fallopian canal"; Archives of Otolaryngology 1946;44:406-08.

16. Kettel K: "Surgery of the facial nerve"; Archives of Otolaryngology 1963;77:327-41.

17. Kodama A, Sando I, Meyers EN, Hashida Y: "Severe middle ear anomaly with underdeveloped facial nerve"; Archives of Otolaryngology 1982;108:93-98.

18. Miehlke A: "Surgery of the facial nerve" Munchen, Urban and Schwarzenberg Verlag; Philadelphia, WB Saunders 1973.

19. Miehlke A, Partsch CJ: "Ohrmissbildung Facialis und Abducenslahmung als Syndromder Thalidomidschadigung"; Arch Ohren Heilk Z Hals Heilk 1963;181:154-74.

20. Nagher GT, Proctor B: "Anatomic variations and anomalies involving the facial canal"; Otolaryngologic Clinics of North America 1991;24(3):531-53.

21. Ombredanne M: "Chirurgie des surdites congenitales par malformation ossicularre"; Annals of Otolaryngology (Paris) 1960;77:423.

❀ ❀ ❀ ❀

Facial expression depends on 7000 motor fibres of the facial nerve firing in unison to bring about muscular contraction. Each of the nerve fibres consists of a central protoplasmic process of parent neuron—the axon which is surrounded by an insulating layer of myelin and by the thin protoplasmic cytoplasm of Schwann cells that constitute the neurilemmal sheath. Around each nerve fibre is a connective tissue tubule, the endoneurium. Many tubules are held together by the perineurium and these bundles are bound together by epineurium (Fig. 2.1).

The facial nerve is highly organized at the CNS level; the degree of topographic organization of the peripheral nerve is controversial. Although clinical observation suggests such a spatial orientation, laboratory investigations demonstrate progressive diffusion and fibre mixing as the nerve courses peripherally.

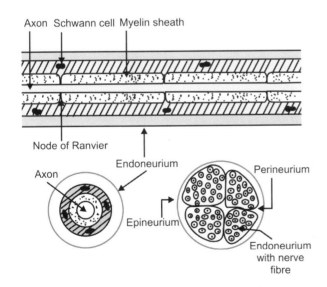

**Figure 2.1**

Diagrammatic representation of a nerve fibre

## DEGREES OF NERVE INJURY

Seddon in 1943 described three types of nerve injury: neuropraxia, axontemesis and neurontemesis.

*Neuropraxia*—Pressure on a peripheral nerve can block the transmission of the impulses without death and degeneration of the axon beyond the site of pressure and may be associated with the loss of myelin at the site of pressure. Release of pressure results in rapid and complete recovery of function without residual deficit. This is a reversible conduction block.

*Axontemesis*—Sectioning of an axon or sufficient pressure to block off axoplasm in the distal segment completely results in the death of the distal segment not at once but after several days.

*Neurontemesis*—Sectioning or disruption of the entire nerve trunk.

After the classification by Seddon, it was Sunderland in 1978 who described five degrees of nerve injury:

- *First degree:* Indicates compression of the nerve that is reversible and the recovery is complete. This is similar to neuropraxic damage to the nerve.
- *Second degree:* There is interruption of the axoplasm and the myelin. This occurs when the compression persists. It results in loss of axons but the endoneurium remains intact. Recovery may take more than 1 to 2 months but is usually complete. This correlates well with the axontemesis type of nerve injury.
- *Third degree:* In the third degree of nerve injury there is loss of myelin tubes due to an increased intraneural pressure. In this case recovery may take as long as 2 to 4 months, there may not be a complete recovery or the recovery though complete may be accompanied by complications of faulty regeneration. The third degree nerve injury correlates with the neurontemesis type of damage.

17

• *Fourth degree:* Fourth degree of nerve injury implies a partial transection of the nerve and recovery is poor.
• *Fifth degree:* In the fifth degree of nerve damage there is a complete transection of the nerve and there is absolutely no recovery.

Thus, by knowing the type of nerve injury it may be possible to assess the prognosis of recovery of the facial nerve function in various disorders. It was found that in Bell's palsy and herpes zoster cephalicus, the first three types of nerve injury were seen. Since the pathological process in these disorders does not progress beyond the first or the second degree the patients usually recover satisfactorily. Partial or complete transection of the nerve is seen more commonly with trauma, tumor or cholesteatoma. In these conditions it is seen how recovery even under ideal conditions is never as good as with the first three degrees of nerve injury.

## NERVE REGENERATION

Nerve regeneration can be defined as a complex interaction of neurons, Schwann cells, extracellular matrix and neurotrophic substances (Selzer, 1987). Regeneration is influenced by various factors and processes. These can be studied by in vivo and in vitro studies. Of the various factors and processes all do not have a clinical application, as they are not very practical. Regeneration follows degeneration, which is usually of the Wallerian type. During regeneration there is sprouting at the axonal end. This is an early process during regeneration and one regenerating axon may produce as many as 20 sprouts. These sprouting ends usually restore the nerve continuity, which is accompanied by reformation of myelin.

Regeneration of the nerve may cause three major changes in the axon: the distance between the node of Ranvier is altered, the myelin covering the axons is much thinner than normal and there is a splitting and crossing of axons that re-innervate the denervated muscle groups without necessarily corresponding to the cell-body unit arrangement that was present prior to degeneraion. This may result in the various compli-

cations of regeneration such as synkinesis, crocodile tears, facial myokimias, hemifacial spasms and stapedius muscle contraction (Schaitkin & May, 1997).

Factors affecting regeneration:
1. *Site of lesion:* Higher the site of the lesion poorer is the prognosis. Closer the lesion to the neuron, poorer is the quality of regeneration.
2. *Duration of the injury:* Longer the duration of the injury, poorer is the prognosis and quality of regeneration.
3. *Age:* Regeneration is better in children than in adults due to a better neural plasticity seen in children.
4. *Nutrition:* A good nutrition is essential for a better functional recovery. Malnourishment deters the process of regeneration.
5. *Blood supply:* Better the blood supply to the injured segment faster is the recovery. Poor blood supply or a compromised blood supply will hamper the chances of regeneration.
6. *Associated injury or infection:* Other associated injuries or infections will produce poorer functional results. The chances of regeneration are poor or nil in an infective bed. Hence, a clean field free from infection is very important for regeneration.

Along with the abovementioned factors, there are certain other biochemical and pharmacological adjuvants that help in the process of regeneration. Though all of them cannot be used in vivo, they provide a promising approach to the regeneration process and may find some use in the future.

### Gangliosides

These agents can be used in vivo for aiding the process of regeneration. Biochemically, gangliosides are complex glycosphingolipids, while functionally they have two properties:
• Neuronotrophic—aiding in survival and maintenance of the neurons
• Neuritogenic—increasing the number and size of branching processes

Gangliosides of bovine origin are commercially available and can be used in peripheral neuropathies.

### Immunomodulators

A nerve injury causes the release of nerve proteins in the blood, which may act as a "foreign antigen." This leads to neuritis and thus hampers regeneration. A similar process may be seen in diseases like amyotrophic lateral sclerosis and Guillain-Barré syndrome.

Also, immunomodulators in the form of immuno-suppressive agents decrease the non-specific inflammation and subsequently fibrosis by limiting the response of macrophages and histiocytes. MacKinnon et al (1987) have found that the immunosuppresssive agents like Azathioprine and Hydrocortisone aid in nerve regeneration.

### Growth Factors

The growth factors important for nerve regeneration include nerve growth factor (NGF) and neurite promoting factor (NPF).

Nerve Growth Factor (NGF) was first described by Levi-Montalcini (Levi-Montalcini & Hamburger, 1953). The peripheral nerve injuries lead to the increased production of NGF.

NGF promotes:
- Increased axonal branching
- Increased dendritic branching
- Prevention of death of neurons

Neurite promoting factor (NPF) has not proven to be of great importance consistently in the process of regeneration. However, it can be considered as a mixture of different growth factors and can be used in certain cases.

### Hormones

ACTH (Strand & Smith, 1980); T3 (Stelmack & Kiernan, 1977); T4 (Danielsen et al, 1986) and Testosterone (Kujawa et al, 1984) have been implicated to increase the rate of regeneration.

## FACIAL NERVE GRADING SYSTEM
### House and Brackmann's Grading System for Recovery of Facial Nerve Function

Approved by 1984 Facial Nerve Disorder Committee of the American Academy of Otolaryngology.

*Grade 1:* Normal

*Grade 2:* Mild dysfunction

Grossly there is a slight weakness noticeable on close inspection, at rest there is normal symmetry and tone. Motion as observed in the forehead is moderate to good, eye closure is complete with slight asymmetry of the mouth.

*Grade 3:* Moderate dysfunction

Grossly there is obvious but no disfiguring difference between two sides and at rest there is normal symmetry and tone. Motion as seen in the forehead is slight to moderate, there is weakness of the angle of the mouth on maximal effort and eye closure is incomplete with maximal effort.

*Grade 4:* Moderately severe dysfunction

Grossly there is obvious asymmetry or disfigurement or both. At rest there may be normal symmetry and tone. There is no motion in the forehead, the eye closure is complete even with maximal effort and there is mouth movement with maximal effort.

*Grade 5:* Severe dysfunction

Grossly there is only barely perceptible motion at rest. Forehead motion is none and eye closure is incomplete and there is very slight mouth movement.

*Grade 6:* Total paralysis, i.e. no movement.

## BIBLIOGRAPHY

1. Danielsen N, Dahlin LB, Ericson LE, et al: Experimental hyperthyroidism stimulates axonal growth in mesothelial chambers. Experimental Neurology 1986;94:54-65.
2. House JW, Brackmann DE: Facial Nerve Grading System. Otolaryngology – Head and Neck Surgery 1985;93:146-47.
3. Kujawa KA, Kinderman NB, Jones KJ: Testosterone induced acceleration from facial paralysis following crush anatomy of the facial nerve in male hamsters. Experimental Neurology 1989;105:80-85.
4. Levi Montalcini R, Hamburger V: A diffusible agent of mouse sarcoma producing hypoplasia of lymphatic ganglia and hyperneurotization of viscera in chick embryos. Journal of Experimental Zoology 1953;123:233-388.

5. MacKinnon SE, Hudson AR, Bain JR, et al: The peripheral nerve allograft: An assessment of regeneration in an immunocompromised host. Plastic and Reconstructive Surgery 1987;79:436-44.

6. Schaitkin B, May M: Disorders of the Facial Nerve. 6th Edition, Scott-Brown's Otolaryngology 1997;3:24/1-38.

7. Seddon HJ: Three types of nerve injury. Brain 1943;66:237-88.

8. Selzer ME: Nerve regeneration. Seminars in Neurology 1987;7:88-96.

9. Strand FL, Smith CM: LPH, ACTH, MSH and motor systems. Pharmacology and Therapeutics 1980;11:509-33.

10. Stelmack BM, Kiernan JA: Effects of Triiodothyronine on the normal and regenerating facial nerve of the rat. Acta Neuropathologica (Berlin) 1977;40:151-55.

11. Sunderland S: Nerve and Nerve Injuries. 2nd Edition. London: Churchill Livingstone: 1978:88-89:96-97;133.

❄ ❄ ❄ ❄

# CHAPTER 3
# Causes of Facial Palsy

## BIRTH

1. Forceps delivery
2. Moebius syndrome
3. Dystrophia myotonica

## TRAUMA

A. Accidental
   1. Skull base fractures
   2. Penetrating injury to middle ear
   3. Barotrauma
   4. Scuba diving
B. Iatrogenic
   1. Mastoid surgery
   2. Parotid surgery
   3. Postaural local anaesthesia
   4. Antitetanus serum
   5. Rabies vaccine
   6. Embolization

## INFECTIONS

A. Bacterial
   1. Malignant otitis externa
   2. Otitis media-acute and chronic with/without cholesteatoma
   3. Tuberculosis
   4. Botulism
   5. Lyme disease
   6. Mastoiditis
B. Viral
   1. Herpes zoster cephalicus (Ramsay Hunt syndrome)
   2 Poliomyelitis
   3. Encephalitis
C. Fungal-Mucormycosis.

## NEOPLASTIC

A. Cerebellopontine angle tumors

1. Vestibular schwannoma
2. Facial nerve tumours
3. Cochlear neuromas
4. Meningioma
5. Ependymoma
6. Arachnoid cyst
B. Temporal bone tumors
   1. Primary
      i. Glomus Jugulare
      ii. von Recklinghausen's disease
      iii. Hans-Schüller-Christian disease
   2. Secondary
      i. Teratoma
      ii. Leukemia
      iii. Sarcoma
C. Parotid tumors
   1. Benign
      i. Pleomorphic adenoma
      ii. Adenolymphoma
      iii. Oxyphil adenoma
   2. Malignant
      i. Mucoepidermoid carcinoma
      ii. Acinic cell carcinoma
      iii. Adenocarcinoma
      iv. Epidermoid carcinoma

## NEUROLOGICAL

1. Opercular syndrome
2. Milliard-Gubler syndrome
3. Encephalitis
4. Multiple sclerosis
5. Myasthenia gravis
6. Charcot-Marie-Tooth disease.

## MISCELLANEOUS

1. Toxic
   i. Tetanus          ii. Diphtheria
2. Metabolic-Diabetes.

❋ ❋ ❋ ❋

*Alok Mohorikar, Vicky Khattar*

## INTRODUCTION

The facial nerve has a complex and tortuous course in the temporal bone and this is where 90% of facial nerve disorders originate (Shambaugh and Clemis, 1973). The testing of the facial nerve becomes important as it helps an otologist to not only evaluate facial palsy but also to treat it at the right time. Facial nerve testing includes not only topognostic tests and prognostic tests but also intraoperative facial nerve monitoring which is gaining significance nowadays and is of surgical interest to the otoneurosurgeons. Many tests have been used to determine the severity and location of facial nerve injury, but controversy still exists with respect to the technique, interpretation and accuracy of the diagnostic tools.

There are various tests, subjective or objective and tests that may or may not use electrical stimulation of the nerve. The intratemporal location of most facial nerve injuries precludes direct assessment of the damaged segment, so facial nerve testing depends upon:

A. Determining the degree of axonal degeneration (Electrodiagnosis)
B. The function of accessory branches (Topognosis)

## Facial Nerve Testing Includes

### Topognostic Tests

1. Lacrimation test (Schirmer's test)
2. Stapedial reflex
3. Salivary flow test
4. Test for the sensation of taste on anterior two-thirds of the tongue
5. Computed tomography.

### Prognostic Tests

1. Electromyography (EMG)
2. Nerve excitibility test (NET)
3. Nerve conduction time
4. Maximal stimulation test (MST)
5. Electroneuronography (ENoG).

### Diagnostic Assessment

1. Blink reflex
2. Electromyography
3. Electroneuronography.

### Intraoperative Monitoring

1. Electrically evoked potential.
2. Mechanically evoked potential.

## Topognostic Tests

They help to determine the site of nerve injury. Not used frequently nowadays because of unreliable information.

### Lacrimal Flow Assessment

Popularised by Tschiassny (1953).

*Schirmer's test:* Lacrimation is studied objectively by Schirmer's test. A strip of filter paper of 5 cm × 0.5 cm is placed in the lower conjunctival fornix of each eye for 5 min and the (soakage) lacrimation of both the sides is compared with inhalation of ammonia to enhance lacrimation. A comparison between the amount of soaked filter paper on the normal and affected side establishes whether there is lessening of tear secretion. A reduction of lacrimation by 30% as compared to the normal side or bilateral reduction to less than 25 mm is considered significant.

### Salivary Flow Test

Introduced by Magielski and Blatt (1958). Techniques include introduction of a No. 50/60 polyethylene catheter in both Wharton's papillae for about 3 mm. The patient is given a few lemon drops to suck for 1 min and the number of drops of saliva over 1 or 5 min is monitored. (Huges, 1989). A 25% reduction between the sides is considered significant.

### Stapedial Reflex

This test provides an advantage of easy and repeated assessment. It is an objective test and eliminates subjective variation and variation in interpretation. Hence, it is commonly called the "Otologist's electromyogram." Koike and colleagues (1977) found that restoration of the stapedial reflex within 3 weeks after onset of facial palsy indicates a functional recovery.

### Taste Sensation (Anterior two-thirds of the Tongue)

This provides useful information in the diagnosis and management of facial palsy and is best assessed by electrogustometry. However, it has not proved to be a useful diagnostic tool.

## Electrodiagnostic Tests

These tests are most reliable prognostic indicators of facial nerve recovery. The tests can be of two types depending upon the direction of the stimulated impulses traveling along the nerve:

- Orthodromic conduction tests: where the nerve is stimulated proximally and muscle response is recorded distally.
- Antidromic conduction tests: where the nerve is stimulated in a retrograde manner. Antidromic tests can detect the nerve injury earlier than Orthodromic tests but have a disadvantage of having multiple artifacts and the responses are difficult to detect.

### Electromyography (EMG)

First used by Weddell and colleagues (1944) for facial paralysis. It measures electric responses during needle insertion, at rest and during volitional movement (Crumley, 1982).

*Possible responses include:*
A. Silent resting potential—indicates normal innervated muscle in a state of rest or severe muscle wasting caused by fibrosis.
B. Voluntary motor unit potential—characterized by triphasic or biphasic morphology with amplitude of 50 to 1500 microvolts.
C. Fibrillation potential—has smaller amplitude and represents involuntary, invisible contraction of a single denervated muscle fibre-indicating degeneration of the muscle nerve supply.
D. Polyphasic re-innervation potential—precedes recovery of denervated muscle fibres and is seen during nerve regeneration.

*Merits of electromyography:*
a. Helps to detect subclinical evidence of early regeneration.
b. Helps to differentiate birth trauma from embryogenic etiology (Harris et al, 1983).
c. Helps in determining the completeness of neural blockade by testing for subclinical voluntary potentials.

*Demerits of electromyography:* However, EMG is not of much use in evaluation of acute paralysis because:
A. 14 to 21 days are required for the development of fibrillation potentials from the time of onset of the facial nerve injury; hence EMG is of use only after14-21 days of nerve injury.
B. Slight electrodental positioning may produce variations in amplitude of response making accurate assessment impossible.

### Nerve Conduction Time (Latency)

This test is similar to evoked EMG in technique. It is used to test the latency response of a muscle (innervated by facial nerve) on electrical stimulation. EMG equipment is used to stimulate the nerve at the stylomastoid foramen and record over one of the facial muscle group such as frontalis (Rogers 1978), mid face (Esselen 1977) or mentalis (Brown et al 1970). The latency for each compound action potential is defined as the time between onset of stimulus and onset of response.

Esselen (1977) and May et al (1974) found this to be the least reliable prognostic test.

### Nerve Excitability Test (NET)

It is most commonly used because it is easy to perform, easily available and it is inexpensive.

Performed by stimulating the nerve at the stylomastoid foramen, and then determining subjectively the presence of a twitch response in the facial musculature. The lowest electric current (threshold) to elicit a facial twitch on the paralyzed side of the face is compared with the threshold value of the normal side. A difference of 3.5-milliampere between sides suggests a poor prognosis.

The main problem with this test is that only large myelinated fibres are stimulated because of their lower threshold, smaller fibres are not recruited until higher thresholds are used and 50% fibres have to be lost before the results are seen. However, it has been seen that despite a normal NET some patients of Bell's palsy had an incomplete recovery.

### Maximal Stimulation Test (MST)

It is best defined as a modified NET, in which maximal rather than minimal stimulation is given to peripheral branches of the facial nerve. The same stimulator is used as in NET with the current set initially at 5 mA and increased to the level of the patient's tolerance. The paralyzed side is compared subjectively to the normal side and is assigned a grade of equal, slightly decreased, markedly decreased or no movement. The latter two responses correlate to a poor prognosis.

### Electroneuronography (ENoG)

Described by Esselen (1977), popularized by Fisch (1981) as electroneuronography (ENoG). May et al (1981) called it as evoked electromyography (EEMG).

It differs from EMG in that bipolar electrodes are used for stimulating as well as recording. Two techniques have been proposed for positioning of electrodes.
  i. Hughes (1981 and 1983) recommends a standard lead placement (SLP)
  ii. Kartush and colleagues (1985) recommended optimized lead placement (OLP).

OLP has shown to be more reliable than SLP and has a better subject tolerence. We have found alae nasi to be an optimum site for lead placement.

After placing the electrodes, the stimulating intensity is gradually increased until smooth biphasic waveform of maximal amplitude is achieved. The response amplitude of the paralyzed side is compared with that of the normal side and the percentage reduction is calculated which correlates most commonly with the axonal degeneration. The rate of amplitude reduction is also correlated with prognosis. Impedance, stimulus amplitude and stimulus frequency affect the response in electroneuronography.

Electroneuronography has been shown to be the most accurate prognostic indicator of all electrodiagnostic tests.

### Magnetic Stimulation

Magnetic stimulation test was first introduced by Barker in 1985 (Barker et al, 1985). Barker stimulated the motor cortex by time varying magnetic fields to induce electrical depolarization. Magnetic fields cause depolarization of the facial nerve at the root entry zone (REZ) by a transcranial penetration. The response can be recorded indirectly by surface electrodes on individual muscles. Magnetic stimulation test shows a longer latency than ENoG as it tests the nerve at a more proximal site, i.e. REZ.

Magnetic stimulation test helps to eliminate the delay in testing nerve function due to its ability to stimulate the intratemporal segment of the facial nerve. Another benefit of magnetic stimulation is the decreased pain in testing compared to electrical stimulation.

### Other Tests

Some of the other tests that can be performed include:
  1. Trigeminofacial (Blink) reflex: This test was first introduced by Overend (1896) by tapping the

glabellar surface. Nowadays it can be done electrically by stimulating the nerve at the supraorbital foramen and recording the EMG response of the orbicularis oculi. The reflex arc in this case uses trigeminal nerve as its afferent and facial nerve as its efferent. It can be considered as a test for the intracranial and the intratemporal portion of the facial nerve.

2. Strength duration curve: This test can be considered as an extension of NET. In this the electrical intensities required for the stimulation of various muscles to evoke contraction is plotted graphically. Depending on their response the degree of axonal degeneration is determined.

## Clinical Application of Electrodiagnostic Tests in Facial Nerve Palsy

- Facial nerve testing provides data, which when combined with the history and physical examination of the patient facilitates adequate counseling and appropriate surgical intervention.
- In patients with poor recovery following Bell's palsy it will help in deciding the exact time for intervention.
- If ENG shows 90% or greater reduction amplitude within 21 days of onset, surgery is indicated.
- ENoG can be used to document the degree of sub-clinical facial nerve involvement and prognosis prior to CP angle and skull base tumor surgery. It also plays a role in the diagnosis of occult tumor involving the facial nerve.
- In managing patients with malignant otitis externa the progression or regression of an underlying neuritis can be monitored by serial ENoG.
- In temporal bone fracture, these tests help in taking decisions about the time of surgery.

## Intraoperative Facial Nerve Monitoring

It is one of the most exciting innovations in ear surgery. The goals of intraoperative monitoring are:
1. Early identification of facial nerve by using electrical stimulation in the soft tissue, tumor or bone.
2. Warning the surgeon of an unexpected facial nerve in the temporal bone or tumor.

3. Mapping the course of the facial nerve in the temporal bone or tumor.
4. Reducing the mechanical trauma to the facial nerve during re-routing or tumor dissection.
5. Evaluation and prognosis of facial nerve function at the conclusion of surgery.

The reasons for use of intraoperative facial nerve monitoring routinely are:
1. The surgeon can judge when it will be needed in a particular case.
2. The operating room personnel become familiar with the equipment.
3. The surgeon learns how to interpret the sounds produced by the monitor and how to correlate them with the surgical manipulation around the facial nerve.

## FACIAL NERVE IMAGING MODALITIES

MRI has supplemented CT as the imaging modality for evaluation of the brain stem, cisternal segment and the intracanalicular segment because:
1. Of superior soft tissue contrast.
2. No change in the position with multiple planes.
3. Interpetrous streak artifacts seen in CT are avoided.

Intravenous administration of Gadolinium—DTPA when combined with T1 weighted imaging sequences increases the sensitivity of acoustic neuroma diagnosis.

## Intratemporal Evaluation of the Facial Nerve

High resolution CT (HRCT) using bone algorithms is the main-stay for evaluating the intratemporal segment. Direct axial and coronal scanning with slice thickness of no more than 2 mm consistently will display the bony labyrinth, facial nerve canal, and the tympanic cavity and its contents. High field strength magnets using standard lead coil and low field strength magnets using a specialized surface now are capable of imaging the facial nerve directly.

## Extratemporal Evaluation of the Facial Nerve

Both MRI and CT scan can be used to demonstrate lesions affecting this segment of the facial nerve. Direct imaging of the facial nerve is possible with MRI. Both CT with contrast and MRI provide the same diagnostic information regarding parotid tumors, it's relationship to facial nerve and it's aggressiveness.

## FACIAL NERVE INJURY/ RECOVERY CLASSIFICATION SYSTEM

### Sunderland's classification of nerve injury describes five degrees of injury (1977):

*Class I*  Neuropaxia.

*Class II*  Axonotmesis.

*Class III*  Disruption of endoneurium.

*Class IV*  Disruption of endoneurium and perineurium.

*Class V*  Neurotemesis.

Electrical testing can distinguish Class I from Class II through V but, cannot make distinction between Classes II through V. The same test results may be obtained from a Class II injury with excellent chances of recovery as from Class V injury with no recovery potential (Sunderland 1978).

***Classification system for reporting results of recovery from facial paralysis (House and Brackmann, 1985).***

This system has been approved and adopted by the Facial Nerve Disorders Committee of the American Academy of Otolaryngology-Head and Neck Surgery, 1984.

| Degree of injury | Grade of recovery | Definition |
|---|---|---|
| 1° (Normal) | I | Normal symmetrical recovery of function. |
| 1°-2° (Mild dysfunction barely noticeable) | II | Slight weakness noticeable only on close inspection |
| 2°-3° (Moderate dysfunction) | III | Obvious weakness but not disfiguring |
| 3° (Moderately severe dysfunction) | IV | Obvious disfiguring weakness with synkinesis, spasm and mass movement |
| 3°-4° (Severe dysfunction) | V | Motion barely perceptible with synkinesis, contracture and absence of spasm |
| Total paralysis | VI | No movement, loss of tone, no synkinesis, contracture or spasm |

## BIBLIOGRAPHY

1. Barker A, Jalinous R, Freeston I: Noninvasive magnetic stimulation of the human motor cortex. Lancet 1985;1:1106-07.
2. Brown E, Arno S, Twedt DC: Bells Palsy. Nerve conduction and recovery time. Physical Therapy 1970;50:799-806.
3. Crumley RL: Electromyography and muscle biopsy in facial paralysis. In: Graham MD, House WF (Eds): Disorders of the Facial Nerve. New York: Raven Press 1982.
4. Esslen E: Electromyography and electroneurography. In: Fisch U (Ed): Facial Nerve Surgery. Birmingham: AL Aesculapius publishing 1977;93-100.
5. Esslen E: Investigations on the localization and pathogenesis of meatolabyrinthine palsies. In: The Acute Facial Palsies New York: Springer-Verlag 1977.
6. Fisch U: Surgery for Bell's palsy. Archives of Otolaryngology 1981;107:1-11.
7. Harris JP, Davidson TM, May M, Thomas F: Evaluation and treatment of congenital facial paralysis. Archives of Otolaryngology 1983;109:145.
8. House JW, Brackmann DE: Facial Nerve Grading System. Otolaryngology—Head and Neck Surgery 1985;93:146-47.
9. Huges G, Nodar R, Williams G: Analysis of test—retest variability in facial electroneurography. Otolaryngology Head and Neck Surgery 1953;91:290-93.
10. Huges G, Josey A, Glasscock M et al: Clinical electroneurography Statistical analysis of controlled measurements in 22 normal subjects. Laryngoscope 1981;91:1834-46.
11. Huges GB: Prognostic tests in acute facial palsy. American Journal of Otolaryngology 1989;10:304-11.
12. Kartush J, Lilly D, Kermink J: Facial electroneurography: Clinical and experimental investigations. Otolaryngology Head and Neck Surgery 1985;93:516-23.
13. Koike Y, Hojo K, Iwasaki E: Prognosis of facial palsy based on the stapedial reflex test. In: Fisch U (Ed): Facial nerve

surgery. Birmingham AL Aesculapius Publishing 1977;159-64.

14. Magielski JE, Blatt IM: Submaxillary salivary flow—a test of chorda tympani nerve function as an aid in diagnosis and prognosis of facial nerve paralysis. Laryngoscope 1958;68:1770-89.

15. May M, Blumenthal F, Klein SR: Acute Bell's palsy: Prognostic value of evoked electromyography, maximal stimulation and other electrical tests. American Journal of Otology 1983;5:1-7.

16. May M, Blumenthal F, Taylor FH: Bell's palsy: Surgery based upon prognostic indicators and results. Laryngoscope 1981;91:2092-2103.

17. Overend W: Preliminary note on a new cranial reflex. Lancet 1896;1:619.

18. Rogers RL: Nerve conduction time in Bell's palsy. Laryngoscope 1978;88:314-26.

19. Shambaugh G, Clemis J: Facial nerve paralysis. In: Paparella M., Shumrick D. (Eds) Otolaryngology: Philadelphia, W.B. Saunders 1973;2:275.

20. Sunderland S: Nerve and Nerve Injuries. 2nd ed. London: Churchill Livingstone 1978;88-89:96-97/133.

21. Tschiassny K: Eight syndromes of facial paralysis and their significance. Annals of Otology, Rhinology and Laryngology 1953;62:677.

22. Weddell G, Feinstein B, Pattle RE: The electrical activity of the voluntary muscle in man under normal and pathologic conditions. Brain 1944;67:178-257.

❀ ❀ ❀ ❀

## INTRODUCTION

Facial nerve is unique among motor nerves. It has a long course through a narrow bony canal called the Fallopian canal. It is due to this that it is more prone to paralysis than any other nerve in the body. The most frequent type of facial palsy is Bell's palsy. Bell's palsy is described as acute idiopathic lower motor neuron palsy of the facial nerve that is usually unilateral, self-limiting, non-progressive, non-life threatening and spontaneously remitting by 4-6 months and always by 1 year. The diagnosis of Bell's palsy is that of exclusion and theoretically it is considered to be accurate only when there is no evidence of any other cause for facial palsy. Nevertheless there is evidence that a typical idiopathic palsy is mediated by a viral inflammatory immune reaction.

Today various modes of treatment have been documented for the management of this condition including medical line of therapy, surgery, and physiotherapy as the understanding of this disease has improved. Thus, it is important for every physician to diagnose this condition and to refer such disease to the otologic surgeon at the earliest remembering the dictum of the celebrated neurologist Gower "A complete unilateral palsy of the face without other symptoms must mean disease of the nerve as it passes through the temporal bone."

## Historical Aspects

In 1829, Sir Charles Bell, an anatomist and a surgeon first described facial palsy and named it "Bell's palsy." He was subsequently knighted for his work. In 1919, Antoni using physical diagnostic techniques labeled the disease as "Acute infectious polyneuritis cerebral acousticofacialis," while in 1960, Dalton identified "Ramsay Hunt syndrome" as a florid form of Bell's palsy.

In 1904, Riek suggested that the cause may be a subclinical middle ear infection and proposed a combined medical and surgical treatment. However, Watermann in 1909 showed that the middle ear was normal in cases of Bell's palsy. There was a divergence of opinion regarding the treatment. In Pietersen's landmark article (Pietersen, 1982), 1101 patients were followed up for a period of one year. It showed that almost 80% of the patients had some return of facial function without any kind of intervention.

The concept of spasm of middle meningeal artery or the stylomastoid artery and paralysis due to ischemia gradually came in. 1950s saw many treatment regimens that included low dose Histamine (Skinner, 1950) to massive doses of Histamine (De Blasio, 1959) and Prednisolone (Taverner, 1954). Korkis (1961) classified patients into two groups—the "vasospastic group" who showed good results with a cervical sympathetic block and the "organic thrombosis group" who did not benefit from the same. Various adjuvants were used like galvanic stimulation, physical therapy—facial support, massage, exercises and splints. They have been recommended and condemned.

For a very long time it was believed that decompression at the stylomastoid foramen was a sufficient treatment for Bell's palsy till Fisch (1977), recommended middle cranial fossa approach to decompress the facial nerve. However, Brackmann felt that decompression of the mastoid portion of the facial nerve was important as the pathology lay there. Transmastoid extralabyrinthine subtemporal approach was described by May in 1979. Thus, at present, we have a number of approaches for decompression of the nerve. However, the role of decompression in cases of Bell's palsy is still debatable.

## Etiology

There are three theories regarding the etiology of Bell's palsy: the vascular ischemia theory, the viral theory and the hereditary theory. Features of each theory support surgical decompression of the facial nerve in selected individuals.

### *Vascular Ischemia Theory*

In the theory of vascular ischemia, the central feature of the pathophysiology is a decrease in the circulation to the facial nerve. Some investigators believe that a primary interruption of one of the major nutrient vessels to the facial nerve is responsible (primary ischemia), but most theorize that the ischemia is secondary to compression of the nerve within the rigid fallopian canal (secondary ischemia). The presence of a thickened fibrous sheath in certain cases causes tertiary ischemia (Grewal et al, 2002) and this theory is recently proposed and elaborated further.

*Primary ischemia:* Vasospasm of the blood vessels leads to the decrease in the blood supply to the facial nerve. Though epineurium has a rich vascular supply, the nerve is relatively avascular due to which primary ischemia will cause a palsy of the nerve.

However, the opponents of this theory cite that the nerve has an adequate blood supply with numerous anastomoses between the stylomastoid and the petrosal blood vessels. Drachmann (1969) has stated that primary ischaemic neuropathy is rare occurring only in certain conditions like the Liereche's syndrome and possibly Diabetes mellitus.

Proponents of this theory have demonstrated lack of significant anastomosis between the stylomastoid and the petrosal vessels (Donath and Lengyel, 1957); decreased vascularity of the horizontal segment of the facial nerve (Blunt, 1954); acute onset facial paralysis following the embolization of the middle meningeal artery (Calcaterra, 1976).

*Secondary ischemia:* Hilger (1949) proposed that the process of primary ischemia leads to secondary ischemia. Hilger described the mechanism of secondary ischemia as follows: The essential features are arteriolar constriction, followed by capillary dilatation with an increase in permeability and resultant transudation. The capillary dilatation may follow ischaemic damage or may result reflexly from a fall in venous pressure. The pressure of fluid transudate is rapidly transmitted to the walls of the lymph capillaries, and they may be closed by compression. Additional fluid then accumulates, and compression of capillaries and venules within the fallopian canal creates further zonal ischemia so that a vicious cycle arises. In severe cases this may lead to necrosis of the nerve, the continuity of which is accordingly interrupted.

This theory of secondary vascular ischemia was the most widely accepted theory for many years. Fundamental investigation of nerve injury has demonstrated that the damaging effect of pressure on nerves is related to blood vessel occlusion rather than to nerve compression alone. Investigators have induced facial paralysis in animals by cold and by constriction of the nerve with a suture and demonstrated histological changes similar to those seen in Bell's palsy. Sunderland (1945) has pointed out the delicate balance of pressures within the fallopian canal that are necessary for continued nutrition of the nerve. Slight swelling that leads to obstruction of venous outflow would then initiate the vicious cycle that results in interference to the arterial blood supply of the nerve.

The cause for the initial swelling within the fallopian canal is not explained. However, it has been theorized that autonomic dysfunction predisposes to vasospasm, but there is no proof for this theory. Mc Govern et al (1966), on the basis of experimental studies, proposed that the triggering mechanism in Bell's palsy is an immunological process of mast cell degranulation, activated by complement or specific allergens. The pathophysiology of edema within the confines of the fallopian canal is the same. The initial vasospasm, increased capillary permeability and edema are due to the histamine release mechanism in immediate hypersensitivity reactions.

According to Fisch (1981), the fundus of the internal auditory meatus is the narrowest portion of the fallopian canal measuring approximately 0.61 mm in diameter while according to Proctor (1991) this narrow segment measures 0.68 mm. This explained why in the presence of edema, the facial nerve fibres (and

29

their vessels) would most often be strangulated at the meatal foramen. The massive bulbous swelling of the meatal segment of the facial nerve occurring in severe cases of Bell's palsy is a typical demonstration of the engagement of the axonal flow, which according to Weiss (1969) is always proximal to the point of pathological constriction of mature nerve fibres.

*Tertiary Ischemia:* In certain longstanding cases of Bell's palsy, the process of secondary ischemia leads to what is called as tertiary ischemia (Grewal et al, 2002). This is because of the presence of a thickened unyielding facial nerve sheath, which has strangulating effect on the nerve and is responsible for residual facial paresis in cases of Bell's palsy (Grewal et al, 2002).

The nerve sheath has three distinct layers—A tough shiny periosteal layer, followed by a layer of loose connective tissue containing blood vessels and a firm layer of fibrous tissue that sends strands that connect the perineural connective tissue. The nerve itself has perineurium, epineurium and endoneurium. The epineurium has a rich vascular supply that communicates freely with the larger vessels. However, the nerve itself is relatively avascular. With this basis of nerve sheath anatomy, the concept of tertiary ischemia can be explained.

In secondary ischemia, the vascular events that take place in the nerve sheath cause vasospasm of the arterioles in the layer of loose connective tissue. This is a temporary reversible event. In most of the cases this temporary vasospasm resolves with complete return of function within 4–6 months. However, in certain cases, it may persist leading to the permanent event of endarteritis of the blood vessels of the nerve sheath. This phenomenon can be demonstrated histologically and is dealt with later in the chapter. Due to this the nerve sheath becomes thickened, fibrous and cordlike. A thicker nerve sheath further enhances the compressive effects on the nerve and it persists even after the resolution of inciting factors. This leads to a permanent residual facial palsy and to prevent this early surgical intervention is required.

## Viral Theory

This theory proposes that Bell's palsy may be a part of polyneuropathy of viral origin. Adour et al (1978)

have found involvement of multiple cranial nerves in cases of Bell's palsy. Also, they have found a stationary titer to Herpes simplex virus or a rising titer to Herpes zoster and also an abnormality in spinal fluid in some patients. Thus, they have concluded that Bell's palsy is an acute benign cranial polyneuritis caused by reactivation of Herpes simplex virus. Djupesland et al (1977) have also proposed that Bell's palsy may be caused due to cranial polyneuropathy that may be viral in origin. This view is supported by May and Hardin (1977) and Tomita (1977) who have also concluded that Herpes simplex or Herpes zoster is a cause of infection. Murakami et al (1996) also reported the involvement of the herpes simplex virus type 1 (HSV-1) in Bell's palsy as a causative agent.

It is proposed that the virus replicates in the ganglion cells causing local damage and hypofunction of the nerves. It then passes down to the axons causing radiculitis. It infects the Schwann cells causing inflammation and autoimmune response. Lymphocytic infiltration follows leading to fragmentation of myelin, demyelination and chromatolysis. When the inflammation and the autoimmune reaction resolve, remyelination follows. Minkowski, in 1891 was the first to provide a careful histological description of the nerve in Bell's palsy. Eight weeks following onset of the palsy, the nerve appeared to be normal from the nucleus to the geniculate ganglion. Distally, within the fallopian canal there were pronounced degenerative Schwann cells. There were no signs of inflammation.

Studies of the nerve sheath by Kettle (1963) and Sade et al (1965) also failed to reveal inflammatory cells. These data would not support an inflammatory etiology for Bell's palsy.

## Hereditary Theory

A familial anatomic variation in the facial canal may account for tendency towards a greater incidence of development of facial palsy later in life. The bony constriction of the fallopian canal leads to acute recurrent attacks of facial palsy. This is commonly seen in osteoporosis group of diseases in which the fallopian canal is of an abnormally small diameter. It also makes the nerve more prone for primary ischaemic insult or viral infections. Kakkar (1966) has concluded this trait of development of recurrent attacks of facial palsy to be a recessive trait.

## Clinical Features

In our experience, the patient usually has a history of exposure to a cold draught of wind as when traveling or a history of splashing cold water on the face followed by pain in the postauricular region which may begin as a deep seated ache and progresses to a severe catch in the upper part of the neck on the ipsilateral side. After a few days the patient notices soap getting into the ipsilateral eye and inability to gargle while washing his/her face in the morning and realizes that there is a facial asymmetry with deviation of the face to the opposite side.

The characteristic features of Bell's palsy are that the facial palsy is usually acute in onset and unilateral with an associated numbness and weakness of the side of the face involved. Some patients may give history suggestive of a viral prodrome or there may be a family history of facial palsy. There may be history of recurrent ipsilateral palsy as well as decreased lacrimation and salivation on the side of the lesion. All patients present with a facial asymmetry with deviation of the face to the opposite side. Almost 90% of the patients show an absent stapedial reflex on impedance audiometry and in some patients the chorda tympani nerve appears red on otoscopic examination within 10 days of onset of the palsy.

The features of presentation in this patient also include upward movement of the eyeball on attempting to close the eye (Bell's phenomenon), epiphora, deviation of the face and the angle of the mouth to the normal side of the face, dribbling of saliva and liquids on attempts to drink, collection of food in the cheek as a result of the paralysis of the buccinator muscle and an inability to blow or whistle. There may be a loss of taste sensation and hyperacusis due to the involvement of the chorda tympani nerve and the stapedius muscle respectively.

However, it is important to know that the classical features of Bell's palsy are that it is "Self limiting, non progressive, non-life-threatening and spontaneously remitting usually within 4-6 months and always by 1 year.

## Histological Aspects

The biopsy of the nerve sheath in cases of Bell's palsy during its surgical decompression shows the presence of endarteritis of the nerve sheath. The microscopic features include the presence of vessels with thickened walls along with a few vessels showing features of obliterative endarteritis. These features are typically seen in cases that have a residual facial palsy.

Also, the other features that can be appreciated are the presence of edema in early cases. In some cases with residual palsy marked amount of fibrosis can be seen in the nerve sheath and thus a thickened nerve sheath is seen microscopically. These typical features can be very well demonstrated by some special stains like the Masson's trichrome which stains the connective tissue green.

## Management of Bell's Palsy

The management of Bell's palsy can be divided into:
1. Medical management.
2. Surgical management.

There exists controversies over what line of treatment should be adopted first and there are various studies, which show the benefit of one over the other. The palsy may be either complete or incomplete when the patient presents to the otologist. It is seen that almost one-third of the patients with incomplete palsy show an evidence of recovery with medical management within three weeks and eventually progress to complete recovery. However, we prefer to start with the medical line of management as soon as the patient presents to us and monitor the progress of the palsy using serial EMG and Nerve Excitability Test repeated every week. Acoustic reflex monitoring is also performed weekly, since it is the first sign of return of nerve function.

## Medical Management

This comprises of high dose steroids (starting with Prednisolone-1 mg/kg/day or 60 mg) given orally in tapering doses over a period of three weeks, Antibiotics, Vasodilators like Xanitol nicotinate, Ascorbic acid, multi-vitamins and vitamin $B_1$, $B_6$ and $B_{12}$, Eye care (eye pad, dark goggles, artificial tears, etc.) and active and passive physiotherapy. Steroids help by providing a protection to the nerve tissue against degeneration of the nerve. Ascorbic acid is known to have antiviral properties. Adour (1991) advocates the use of Acyclovir orally in the dose of 200 to 400 mg five times per day.

The medical treatment forms the main stay of Bell's palsy and it results in improvement of most of the cases. However, if signs of recovery fail to appear within three weeks of medical management, we advocate surgical decompression of the nerve.

## Surgical Treatment

This includes the decompression of the facial nerve that may be done by various approaches. They include middle cranial fossa approach; translabyrinthine approach; transmastoid extralabyrinthine subtemporal approach and total decompression that may be a combination of the approaches mentioned above.

It still remains controversial whether a case of Bell's palsy should be offered surgical treatment and at what point of time should it be offered. There are no strict criteria so as to when the facial nerve should be decompressed. Various researchers have debated on the role of surgical decompression. The Marsh and Coker criteria (1991) state the following indications:
• Complete denervation
• Paralysis for more than 4-6 weeks
• Incomplete return of function in 60 days
• Recurrent facial palsy
• Nerve excitability test shows a difference of 3.5 mA on both the sides

Schirmer's test can be used to decide the mode of surgical decompression—if the tear flow is reduced by more than 50% on the affected side then a total decompression or middle fossa approach is indicated.

We advocate facial nerve decompression in a case of Bell's palsy if there is no improvement of the palsy after 3 weeks of medical treatment or if the palsy appears to be progressively worsening inspite of the patient being on medical management. Facial nerve decompression can be carried out for a patient presenting upto 2 years after onset of palsy. However, if a patient presents after 2 years of onset of palsy, regeneration usually does not occur and plastic surgical repair has to be considered.

It is known that in a case of Bell's palsy, the facial nerve shows "skip lesions", i.e. segments of normal nerve tissue in between areas of pathology. Keeping this in mind, we prefer a complete/total decompression of the nerve, this includes decompression of labyrinthine, tympanic, and mastoid segments till the stylomastoid foramen.

We carry the decompression of the facial nerve through a transmastoid approach via a posterior tympanotomy. A standard postauricular incision is taken with an anteriorly based pedicled flap. A complete cortical mastoidectomy is done and a posterior tympanotomy is performed. The mastoid segment of the facial nerve is then decompressed. The incus is disarticulated, if necessary and temporarily translocated in the middle ear. The middle fossa dura is then skeletonised and the decompression proceeded proximal to the second genu till the entire nerve is decompressed (Figs 5.1a to c and 5.2 a and b).

During facial nerve decompression, we have seen that the nerve sheath in a case of Bell's palsy appears unusually thickened due to fibrosis (Figs 5.3 a to d). This is an important factor in creating a vicious cycle of further compressing the edematous nerve resulting in tertiary ischemia due to the compressive effects of the rigid thickened nerve sheath, even after removing the compression caused by the bony facial canal in addition to secondary ischemia due to a rigid bony fallopian canal and worsening of the edema. Hence, we prefer to slit the nerve sheath and relieve the nerve of the strangulating effects of the nerve sheath. Also, we have seen varying pictures of nerve pathology after the sheath is slit and depending on these, we start postoperative treatment (Fig. 5.4). The pathologies seen include: an edematous nerve, where we start steroids postoperatively; a congested nerve where we start Acyclovir in addition to steroids postoperatively or a thinned out atrophic nerve due to fibrosis as a result of disuse atrophy.

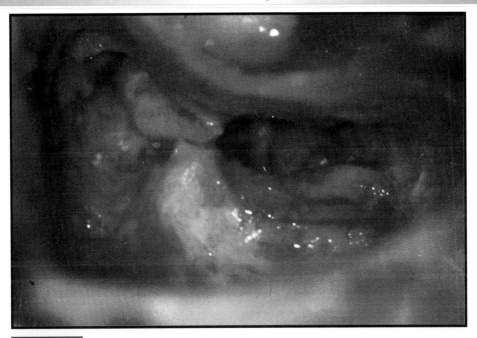

**Figure 5.1 a**

Intraoperative photograph showing facial nerve decompression through a posterior tympanotomy in a patient of Bell's palsy. Note the markedly edematous nerve bulging through the slit nerve sheath

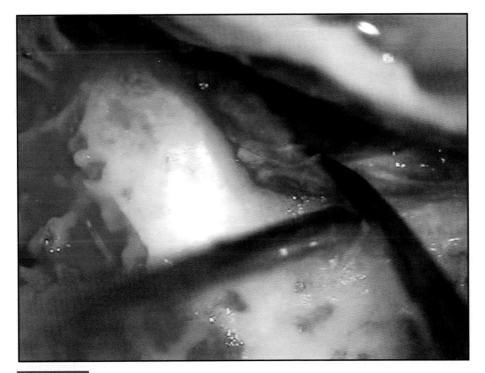

**Figure 5.1 b**

A case of long-standing Bell's palsy (18 weeks duration) where decompression of the nerve, with slitting of it's sheath revealed multiple sites of nerve compression due to fibrous bands which were cut

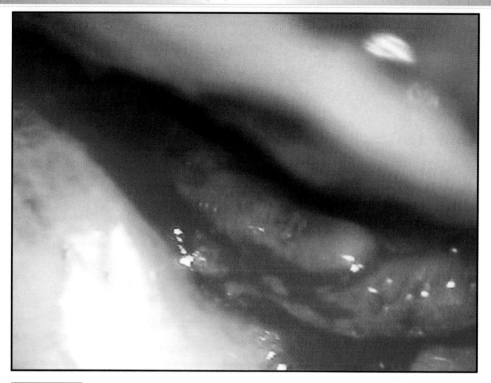

**Figure 5.1 c**

The decompressed nerve with severe oedema and multiple indentations due to the compressive effect of the fibrous bands even after they were cut. The nerve is seen bulging out of the cut sheath

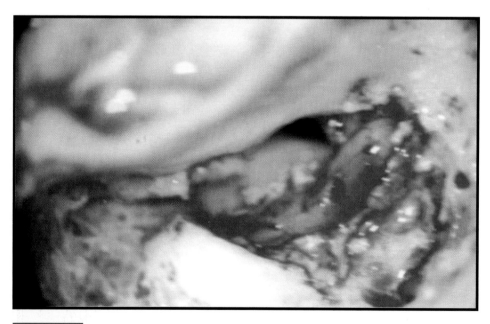

**Figure 5.2 a**

Intraoperative photograph of the facial nerve decompressed in a case of Bell's palsy with slitting of its sheath

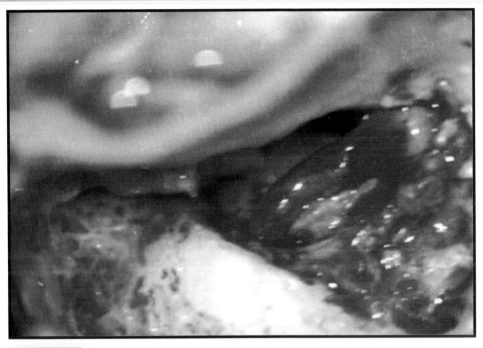

**Figure 5.2 b**

Intraoperative photograph of the facial nerve decompressed in a case of Bell's palsy. The nerve is seen removed from its sheath. Note the edema at the stylomastoid foramen

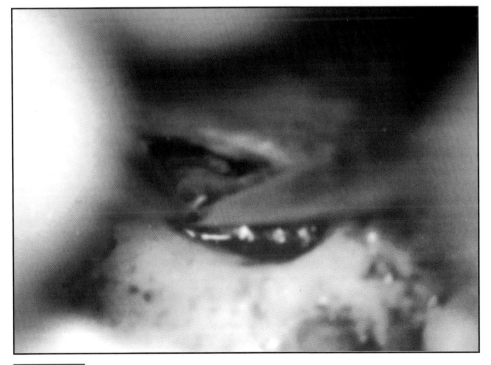

**Figure 5.3 a**

Intraoperative photograph showing the fibrosed and thickened facial nerve sheath in a decompression done for a case of Bell's palsy—a biopsy of its sheath being taken

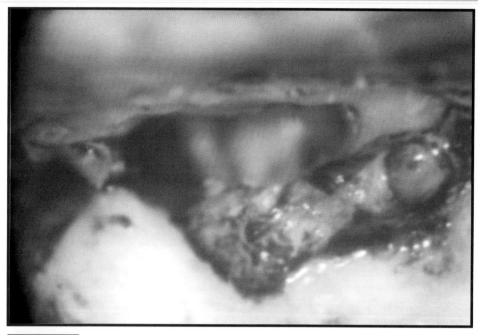

**Figure 5.3 b**

Intraoperative photograph showing the fibrosed and thickened facial nerve sheath in decompression done for a case of Bell's Palsy-Biopsy taken—note the nerve bulging out through the biopsy site

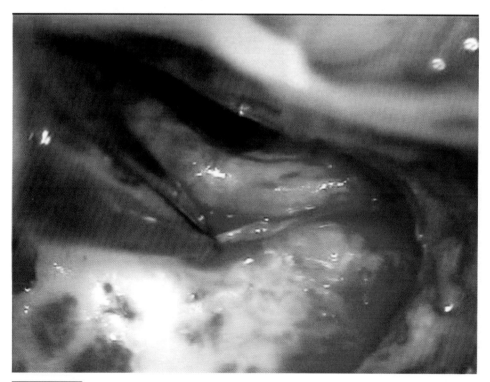

**Figure 5.3 c**

Intraoperative photograph of facial nerve decompression in another case of Bell's palsy, its sheath is caught with forceps for taking biopsy

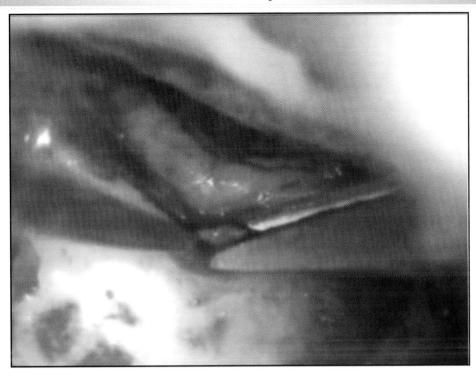

**Figure 5.3 d**

Intraoperative photograph of facial nerve decompression in the same case of Bell's palsy where biopsy of the thickened and fibrosed nerve sheath is being taken

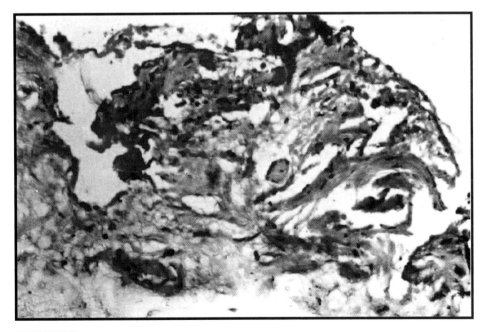

**Figure 5.4**

Histopathology of the facial nerve sheath showing bundles of facial nerve fibres with intervening fibrosis (H&E staining 20X) of the same patient (Figs 5.3 c and d)

There are certain unique anatomical and surgical factors, which if considered during the procedure make the operation much simpler.

### Anatomical Factors

A thorough knowledge of the anatomy of the antrum threshold angle (Mihalkovics, 1892) and chorda facial angle (Plester, 1965) is important before performing the posterior tympanotomy. However, we have noticed certain important anatomical facts that will aid the surgeon in performing a posterior tympanotomy:

1. The posterior canal wall takes a gentle natural curve in its deep part, an anatomical fact that aids a surgeon in performing a posterior tympanotomy. A simple mastoidectomy is performed and the posterior meatal wall is thinned as much as possible. After this the opening of the facial recess can be commenced. To locate the site of opening of the facial recess, a straight line is drawn parallel to the posterior canal wall at the 3 O'clock position. This line will fall on the facial nerve in its mastoid segment. Also, due to this natural curve of the deep part of the external auditory canal, the chorda tympani lies more anteriorly and the facial nerve lies posteromedially. The removal of the bone between the chorda and this straight line will open the facial recess.

2. The facial nerve, in its mastoid segment, takes a gentle turn anteriorly as it approaches the stylomastoid foramen. This is a consistent feature found in all the cases and we have termed this as the ***third genu of the facial nerve*** (Fig. 5.5). This peculiar anatomical course of the facial nerve defines the lower limit of posterior tympanotomy. During surgery, if an imaginary line is drawn from the floor of the middle ear in the antero-posterior axis, the third genu begins at the point where this line meets the facial nerve. The third genu starts in the mastoid segment of the facial nerve and continues in its extratemporal portion. We feel that the facial nerve should be identified by the third genu itself near the area of its exit through the stylomastoid foramen as it forms a consistent landmark. This, if identified can be considered as

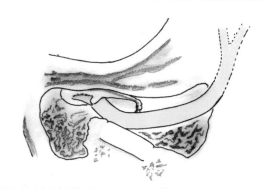

**Figure 5.5**

Diagrammatic representation of the third genu of the facial nerve

a more reliable landmark than the more conventional landmarks for the facial nerve in this region viz. the digastric ridge in its mastoid segment and the Tragal pointer in its extratemporal segment.

### Surgical Factors

The following surgical factors are very useful during posterior tympanotomy in our experience:

1. Posterior tympanotomy is a very simple procedure as it as a mere extension of a simple mastoidectomy. After completing a cortical or simple mastoidectomy, the posterior canal wall is thinned and the facial recess opened. The posterior tympanotomy finally assumes a bean shaped opening in the posterior canal wall. However, with the standard surgical position of the patient, this bean shaped opening gives a limited view of the middle ear structures. This difficulty can be eliminated by tilting the head of the patient downward, i.e. away from the operating surgeon. This will apparently increase the working distance and thus the area under vision. In such a position, the chorda tympani and the facial nerve lie in approximately the same horizontal plane, which lies perpendicular to the visual axis of the surgeon. As a result, certain important middle ear structures such as the tympanic part of the facial nerve, the eustachian tube opening and the hypotympanum

are now clearly visible and easily accessible. We have termed this as *the open window effect* (Figs 5.6 a and b).

2. The posterior tympanotomy can be extended superiorly upto the 12 O'clock position or a little beyond anteriorly and hence the term *postero-superior tympanotomy* appears more appropriate when used in this context.

Therefore, although some may not advocate surgical decompression in a case of Bell's palsy, we prefer decompression provided there is a definite indication for the same. If indicated, we feel that transmastoid decompression is a safe and an easy approach to decompress the entire facial nerve and the above-mentioned factors should be considered by an otologic surgeon to facilitate the procedure of decompression via posterior tympanotomy.

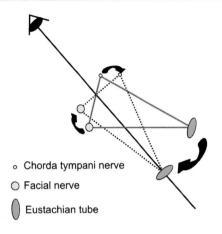

o Chorda tympani nerve

○ Facial nerve

Eustachian tube

**Figure 5.6 a**

Diagrammatic representation showing tilting of the patient's head away from the surgeon, bringing the chorda tympani nerve and the facial nerve in a horizontal plane, perpendicular to the surgeon's visual axis, thus improving visibility— "open window effect"

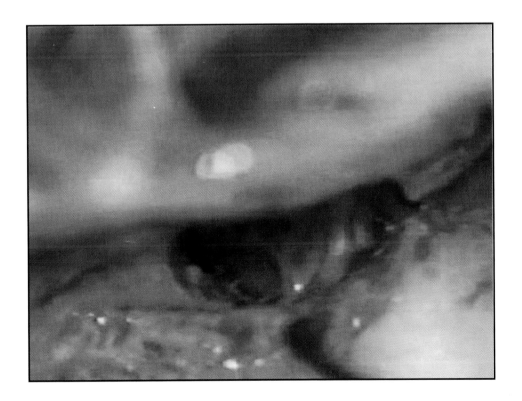

**Figure 5.6 b**

Improved visibility of structures through a posterior tympanotomy on tilting the patient's head away from the surgeon— "open window effect"

## BIBLIOGRAPHY

1. Adour KK: Medical Management of Idiopathic (Bell's) Palsy. The Otolaryngologic Clinics of North America 1991;24:663-72.

2. Adour KK, Byl FM, Hilsinger RL et al: The true nature of Bell's palsy: Analysis of 1000 Consecutive Patients. Laryngoscope 1978;89:787-801.

3. Blunt MJ: The Blood supply of the Facial nerve. Journal of Anatomy 1954;888:520.

4. Calcaterra TC, Rand RW, Bentson JR: Ischaemic Paralysis of Facial Nerve: A Positive Etiological factor in Bell's palsy. Laryngoscope 1976;86:92-97.

5. Dalton GA: Bell's palsy: Some Problems of Prognosis and Treatment. British Medical Journal 1960;1:1765-70.

6. Donath T, Lengyel I: The vascular structure of the intrapetrosal section of the facial nerve, with special reference to peripheral facial palsy. Acta Med Acad. Sci Hung. 1957;10:249.

7. Djupesland G, Berdal P, Johannessen JA et al: Viral infection as a cause of acute peripheral facial palsy. Archives of Otolaryngology 1976;102:403-06.

8. Drachman D: Bell's Palsy—A Neurological point of view. Archives of Otolaryngology, 1969;89:147.

9. Fisch U: Surgery For Bell's palsy. Archives of Otolaryngology 1981;107:1-11.

10. Grewal DS, Hathiram BT, Walvekar R, Mohorikar AV, Shroff M, Bahal NK: Surgical Decompression in Bell's palsy—Our viewpoint. Indian Journal of Otolaryngology and Head and Neck Surgery 2002;54:198-203.

11. Hilger JA: The nature of Bell's palsy. Laryngoscope, 1949;59:228.

12. Kettel K: Pathology and surgery of Bell's palsy. Laryngoscope 1963;73:837.

13. Korkis FB: Treatment of Recent Bell's palsy by Cervical sympathetic block. Lancet 1961;1:255-57.

14. Marsh MJ, Coker NJ: Surgical Decompression of Idiopathic Facial Palsy. Otolaryngologic Clinics of North America, 24:675-90.

15. May M, Hardin WB: Facial Palsy: Interpretation of Neurological Findings. (Trans.) Am Acad Ophthalmol Otol: 84: ORL 1977;710-22.

16. May M: Total Facial Nerve Exploration: Transmastoid, Extralabyrinthine, Subtemporal: Indication and Results. Laryngoscope 1976;89:906.

17. McGovern FH, Thompson E, Link N: The experimental production of ischaemic facial paralysis. Laryngoscope, 1966;76:1138.

18. Mihalkovics G: The Morphology of the Central Nervous System and Sensory Organs. (Hungarian) Franklin Co., Budapest; 1892.

19. Minowski: Zur pathologischen Anatonnie der rhurriatischen Facialislahmung. Archives of General Psychiatry 1891;23:586.

20. Murakami S, Mizobuchi M, Naakaashiro Y et al: Bell's palsy and Herpes Simplex Virus: Identification of Viral DNA in Endoneural fluid and Muscle. Annals of Internal Medicine 1996;124:27-30.

21. Proctor B: The Anatomy of the Facial Nerve. Otolaryngologic Clinics of North America 1991;24:479-529.

22. Peiterson E: The Natural History of Bell's palsy. American Journal of Otology 1982;4:107-111.

23. Plester (1965). Cited by Jako CJ: The posterior route to the middle ear: Posterior tympanotomy, Laryngoscope 1967;77:306-16.

24. Sade J, Levy E, Chaco J: Surgery and pathology of Bell's palsy. Archives of Otolaryngology 1965;82:594.

25. Schaitkin B, May M: Disorders of the facial nerve. 6th edition Scott – Brown's Otolaryngology 1977;3:24/1-38.

26. Seddon HJ: Three types of nerve injury. Brain 1943;66:237-88.

27. Sunderland S: Blood supply of the peripheral nerves. Archives of Neurology and Psychiatry 1945;54:280.

28. Sunderland S: Nerve and Nerve Injuries. 2nd edition. London: Churchill Livingstone 1978;88-89,96-97,133.

29. Taverner D: Lancet 1954;2:1052.

30. Tomita H: In Facial Nerve Surgery Ed. By U. Fisch Amsterdam, Kugler Medical Publication, 1977.

31. Weiss PA: Neuronal dynamics and neuroplasmic ('axonal') flow. New York: Academic Press, 1969;8.

32. William Gowers as cited by: Cawthorne, T and Wilson, T "Indications of Intratemporal Facial Nerve Surgery", Archives of Otolaryngology, 1963;78:429-34.

❊ ❊ ❊ ❊

# CHAPTER 6

# Facial Palsy in Infection

Intratemporal lesions are by far the most common cause of facial paralysis. In a series of 322 cases, Cawthorne found that 8% (26 patients) were due to chronic otitis media. Of all cases of otitis, 1% (Tonndorf 1924), 1.8% (Lund 1929) or 2% (Kettel 1943) show a facial palsy.

The various infections, which can cause facial palsy, include:

1. Acute suppurative otitis media.
2. Acute mastoiditis.
3. Chronic suppurative otitis media.
   i. Cholesteatoma.
   ii. Granulations.
   iii. Tuberculous otitis media.
   iv. Aural polyp.
   v. Tympanosclerosis.
4. Malignant otitis externa.
5. Herpes zoster oticus.
6. Otogenic abscesses.
   i. Citelli's abscess.
   ii. Luc's abscess.
   iii. Bezold's abscess.

## Acute Suppurative Otitis Media (A.S.O.M) and Acute Mastoiditits

Facial palsy can occur secondary to A.S.O.M and acute mastoiditits, if the treatment is inadequate or if the organisms are very virulent or if the host immunity is low. This is commonly seen in children.

In acute otitis media, particularly in children early facial palsy is seen occasionally (0.5% Vogt 1899, Kettel 1943). Such early paralysis is thought to be due to toxic neuritis (Lund 1929), a collateral hyperemia (Burger 1925) or edema of the loose fibrous tissue of the nerve. According to Pollack (1928), this edema may be due to a toxic vasomotor paresis of the epineural vessels. It has been assumed, not without controversy (Fremel 1931, Lange 1917) that toxins may reach the nerve via dehiscence in the fallopian canal (Nuhsmann 1926, Mayer 1932) or via the fine bony canals of the chorda tympani and the stapedius nerve (Rudinger1932, Sade 1965).

The cause of facial palsy in A.S.O.M is usually due to severe infection affecting the facial nerve in the presence of congenital dehiscences of the fallopian canal, usually in its tympanic segment.

The palsy usually responds well to antibiotics and myringotomy with a complete recovery. Rarely, a surgical decompression may be required in the presence of a coalescent mastoiditis.

## Chronic Suppurative Otitis Media

### Cholesteatoma

Facial palsy is 3-4 times more common in cholesteatoma than in A.S.O.M. The facial palsy that occurs in a cholesteatoma is due to the erosion of the fallopian canal by the cholesteatoma matrix (Figs 6.1 a and b) following which the palsy is caused due to direct pressure on the nerve and the effect of various enzymes secreted by the cholesteatoma matrix. Involvement of the facial nerve is directly proportional to the size and extent of the cholesteatoma, which determines the intensity of infection, which is responsible for the palsy. A number of cases have been described in which the intact nerve ran freely through the tympanum and the substance of the cholesteatoma (Lund 1929, Kettel 1943). This seems to indicate that the real cause of facial palsy in such cases is compression, which is caused by inflammatory edema of the neurilemma (Eisinger 1925, Hall 1941, Lund 1929, Neumann 1906, Pollman 1937) and by hyperemia and serous infiltration of the endosteum (Krischek 1950, Neumann

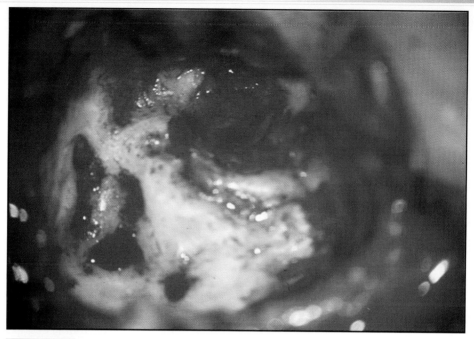

**Figure 6.1 a**

Tympanomastoid surgery with an exposed facial nerve as seen after removal of the cholesteatoma matrix. The edges of the eroded fallopian canal are ragged, due to the disease process

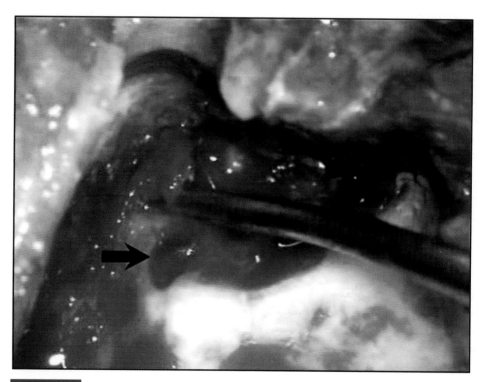

**Figure 6.1 b**

A case of labyrinthine fistula covered by a bony sequestrum. The patient also had facial nerve palsy

1906). Kettel emphasized that in his opinion it is not so much direct pressure on the axons but strangulation of epineural vessels, which produces paralysis. Postmortem findings of Darkeschewitsch (1893) as well as Flatau (1897), confirm this view.

Treatment is by decompression of the nerve with removal of the matrix which drapes over the dehiscent nerve as it can be easily peeled off from the nerve sheath.The various methods by which the matrix can be peeled off include peeling it using a suction and sickle knife, gently peeling it off using a moist cotton ball or as we advocate, irrigating the cavity with water/saline which results in the floating of the edges of the matrix which now is easily demarcated and then removed by suction and instrumentation. The outer layer of the nerve sheath is relatively thick because it is the periosteal layer and hence it offers protection to the nerve against infection and instrumentation. Antibiotics with steroids both locally as well as systemically are given post-operatively for ten days.

### Granulations

They tend to erode the bone of the fallopian canal and affect the bare nerve resulting in facial palsy.

### Tuberculous Otitis Media

It usually presents with complications of C.S.O.M. such as facial palsy, labyrinthitis secondary to labyrinthine fistula, meningitis and intracranial abscess (Grewal and Hathiram 1999). Facial palsy tends to occur early in tuberculous otitis media due to erosion of bone by the granulation tissue and formation of bony sequestra (Ormerod, 1931) (Fig. 6.1b). In advanced/late cases there may be a huge tuberculoma in the mastoid causing facial palsy (Figs 6.2 a and b).

Treatment consists of decompression of the facial nerve with removal of granulations and the bony sequestra, which may press upon the nerve, followed by antituberculous therapy.

### Aural Polyp

Occasionally, an aural polyp may be adherent to a dehiscent facial nerve in its tympanic segment and on attempting to remove this polyp there may be facial twitching which should alert the surgeon to this possibility. Therefore, in such cases a polypectomy and mastoidectomy are planned as one-stage surgery (Fig. 6.3).

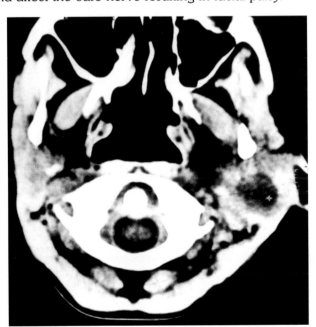 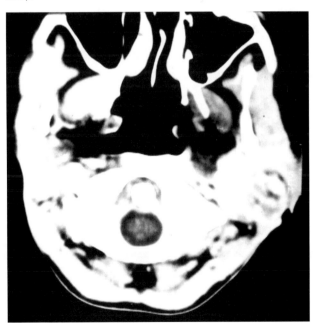

**Figures 6.2 a and b**

CT scan showing presence of a heterogenous space occupying lesion in the temporal bone resulting in widening of the temporal bone. Histopathology revealed it to be a tuberculoma. (a) Plain, (b) Contrast showing enhancement

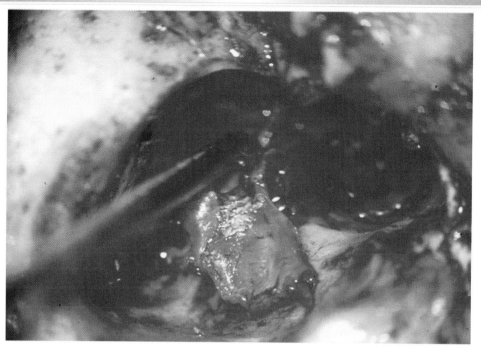

**Figure 6.3**

A polyp of tuberculous origin arising from the fallopian canal. In this case, manipulation of the polyp resulted in facial twitchings hence a canal wall down mastoidectomy was performed for removal of polyp and clearance of the mastoid air cell system

### Tympanosclerosis

The tympanic cavity and the fallopian canal are common sites of tympanosclerosis. A tympanosclerotic plaque may be rarely adherent to a dehiscent facial nerve in its tympanic and/or labyrinthine segment and removal of tympanosclerosis from the attic region during surgery should be undertaken with due precaution to prevent damage to a dehiscent facial nerve. However, there is no pathology seen in the facial nerve in cases of tympanosclerosis (Fig. 6.4).

### Malignant Otitis Externa

Pseudomonas infection generally seen in debilitated or elderly and uncontrolled diabetics that begins in the external auditory canal to progressively involve the temporal bone and skull base is termed as malignant otitis externa. This infection is often associated with facial paralysis, due to bone erosion. Treatment is by extensive surgical debridement and antibiotics with steroids as well as control of diabetes mellitus.

### Herpes Zoster Oticus: (Ramsay Hunt Syndrome) (Fig. 6.5)

This is a multicranial nerve involvement by the herpes zoster virus. Typically the individual manifests with sudden onset facial paralysis associated with severe pain in the ear and mastoid region. The auricle and external auditory meatus are inflamed and red with painful vesicles filled with clear fluid. The facial palsy is probably due to edema of the nerve particularly in the area of the geniculate ganglion. Treatment is non-surgical usually with Acyclovir orally 800 mg 3-5 times a day for 5 days.

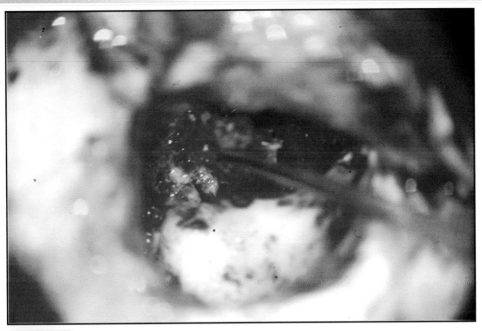

**Figure 6.4**

Intraoperative photograph of tympanomastoid surgery showing a large plaque of tympanosclerosis which was covering the eroded fallopian canal and involving the facial nerve in its tympanic segment. The patient did not have facial palsy

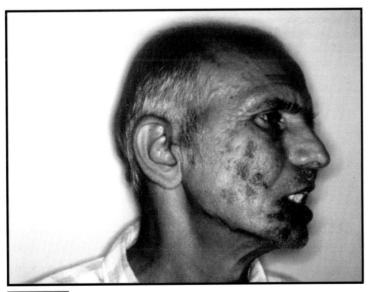

**Figure 6.5**

Clinical photograph of a patient of herpes zoster oticus with facial palsy

## Otogenic Abscesses

Extracranial abscesses such as Bezold's, Citelli's and Luc's abscesses secondary to unsafe C.S.O.M (Tuberculous otitis media, cholesteatoma or granulations) cause facial palsy due to erosion of bone with necrosis of the fallopian canal, in the region of the stylomastoid foramen in case of Bezold's abscess and in the mastoid segment due to Luc's abscess or a Citelli's abscess. The facial palsy is probably due to both necrosis of bone of the fallopian canal as well as severe infection and inflammation of the facial nerve (Figs 6.6 to 6.8).

45

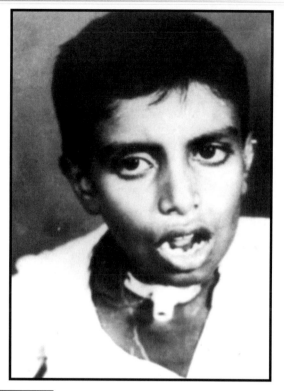

**Figure 6.6 a**

An 8-year old boy 4 days after draining of parapharyngeal space abscess (Citelli's) with marked cellulitis of the neck

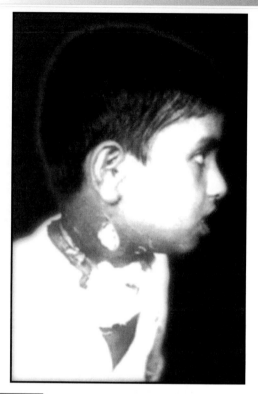

**Figure 6.6 b**

Same patient (Figure 6.6a) lateral view showing ear discharge and gauze pack in the drained abscess cavity

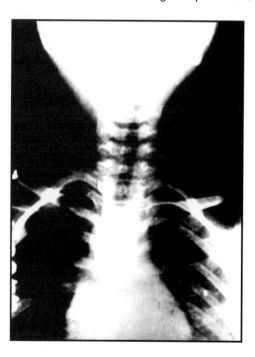

**Figure 6.6 c**

X-ray of the neck and chest of the same patient (Figure 6.6a)showing soft tissue shadow on right side of the neck with marked shift of trachea to the left

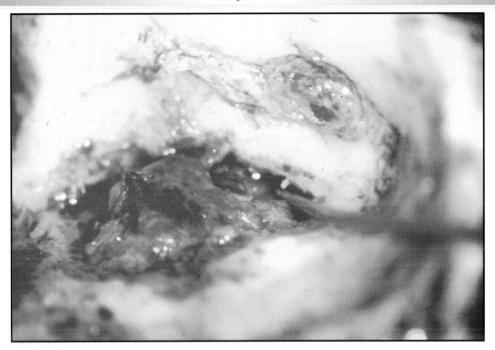

**Figure 6.6 d**

Radical mastoidectomy cavity of the same patient (Fig. 6.6a). Note the cavity eroded at its base by tuberculous granulation tissue and the pick in the fistulous track under the exposed digastric muscle, which resulted in pus entering the parapharyngeal space to cause a Citelli's abscess

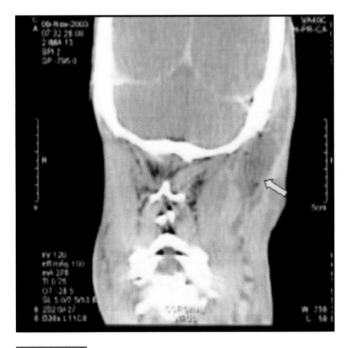

**Figure 6.6 e**

Coronal CT scan showing Citelli's abscess in another patient

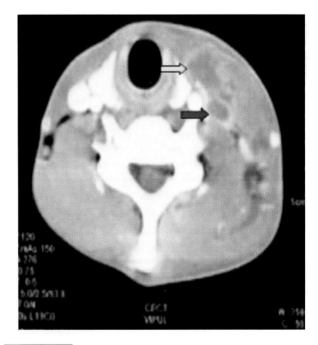

**Figure 6.6 f**

Axial CT scan of same patient (Figure 6.6 e) showing Citelli's abscess with internal jugular vein thrombosis

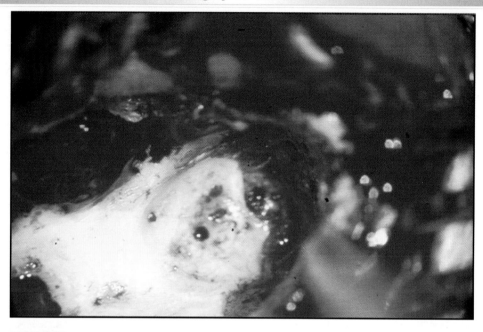

**Figure 6.7**

Intraoperative photograph of tympanomastoid surgery in a case of Bezold's abscess. The entire bony tip is eroded by disease process including the stylomastoid foramen. This was tuberculous in origin as diagnosed from the histopathology report of granulation tissue

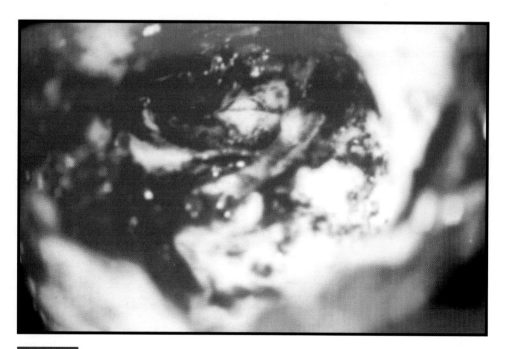

**Figure 6.8**

Intraoperative photograph showing Luc's abscess of tuberculous origin. This patient presented with facial palsy

## BIBLIOGRAPHY

1. Burger H: Lahmung des Gesichtsnerven bei akuter Mittelohrentzundung. Ndld. Tschr. Geneesk. 1925, quoted from Pollak.
2. Darkeschewitsch L: Zur Frage von den pathologisch-anatomischen Veranderungen bei peripherer Facialislahmung nicht spezifischen Ursprungs Neur Zbl. 1893;12:329.
3. Eisinger K : Bezoldmastoiditis mit Facialislahmung in allen drei Asten Mschr Ohrenhk 1925;59:863.
4. Flatau E: Peripherische Facialislahmung mit retrograder Neurondegeneration; ein Beitrag zu der normalen und pathologischen Anatomie der Nn. facialis, cochlearis und trigeminus. Z Klin Med 1897;32:280.
5. Fremel F: Zur Pathologie der otogenen Gesichtslahmung. Mschr Ohrenhk 1931;65:950.
6. Grewal DS, Hathiram BT: "Tuberculous Otitis Media" in ENT Disorders in a tropical Environment 2nd ed published by MERF publications and Edited by Prof. S. Kameswaran and Prof. Mohan Kameshwaran (1999), Chennai, India 65-77.
7. Hall A: Pathology of Bell's palsy. Archives of Otolaryngology. Am 1941;54:475.
8. Kettel K: Facial palsy of otitic origin. Arch. Oto-laryng (Am) 37( 1943), 303.Ormerod, F.C " Tuberculous disease of the middle ear" Journal of Laryngology and Otology 1931;46:449-59.
9. Krischek J: Facialislahmung und Poliomyelitis. Arztl Wschr 1950;6:421.
10. Lange W: Pathologie der Taubstummheit. In: MANASSE: Handbuch der pathologischen Anatomie des menschlichen Ohres, Bergmann, Wiesbaden 1917.
11. Lund R: Die Facialisparese bei den suppurativen Mittelohrleiden mit besonderem Hinblick auf ihre Verbindung mit labyrintharen Komplikationen and ihre Bedeutung als Operationsindikation. Z. Hals-usw. Hk. 1929;23:296.
12. Mayer O: Quoted from Szende. Szende, B.: Herpes zoster oticus mit Facialislahmung. Mschr Ohrenhk1932;66:814.
13. Neumann H: Die otitischen Facialisparesen. Wien. Med. Wschr. 1906;56:1233/1306-355.
14. Nuhsmann T: Diagnose, Prognose und Therapie der otogenen Facialislahmung. In: Handbuch der Hals-Nasen-Oherenheilkunde vii/2 Bergmann, Munchen; Springer: Berlin 1926.
15. Ormerod F C: "Tuberculous disease of the middle ear".
16. Pollak E: Affektionen im Gebiete des Trigeminus und Facialis,In: Alexander und Marburg: Handbuch der Neurologie des Ohres ii/I. Urban and Schwarzenberg, Berlin-Wien 1928.
17. Pollmann L: Facialisparesen. Mschr. Ohrenhk 1937;71:1068.
18. Rudinger: quoted from SZENDE: Herpes zoster oticus mit Facialislahmung. Mschr. Ohrenhk 1932;66:814.
19. Sade J: Retrograde facial paralysis. Annals of Otology (St. Louis) 1965;74:94.
20. Tonndore W: Facialiskrampfe. Z Hals-usw Hk 1924;8:98.
21. Vogt H: Die Paralyse des Nervus facialis im Anschlub an Otitis media acuta; ein Beitrag von derLehre der otogenen Gesichtslahmung. Dissertation Heidelberg 1899 (quoted from Pollack).

❋ ❋ ❋ ❋

# CHAPTER 7
# Facial Nerve in Temporal Bone Fractures

## INTRODUCTION

The human race today faces an uncontrolled and mounting epidemic of severe injuries and death due to trauma. Since direct trauma to the ear in closed head injuries constitutes a major cause of correctable ear pathology, a particular discussion of fractures of the temporal bone desires the readers' closest attention. (Hough and Stuart, 1968).

Temporal bone fractures are extremely common with head injuries. They present with a variety of symptoms including facial nerve paralysis, hearing loss, vertigo and leakage of the CSF through the ear or the nose. Since the temporal bone is the domain of the otologist, he plays a major and important role in management of fractures along with the neurosurgeon.

Fractures involving the temporal bone can be classified depending on the relationship of the fracture line to the long axis of the petrous part of the temporal bone as: Longitudinal, Transverse and Mixed (Fig. 7.1).

The facial nerve is rendered functionless either temporarily or permanently in longitudinal fractures whereas the risk of permanent facial nerve palsy is much more in transverse fractures. Kettel (1950) believed that an immediate paralysis should be explored as soon as the patient's condition permits.

The facial nerve paralysis could be due to:
- An incomplete or complete transection of the nerve
- Bony fragments compressing on the nerve
- Edema of the nerve as a part of generalized inflammation due to trauma
- Compression due to the bands formed in the nerve sheath which is caught between the fractured fragments.

Often the diagnosis is made purely on clinical grounds as the fractures are not always seen on routine skull X-rays. Rarely the diagnosis is delayed until the

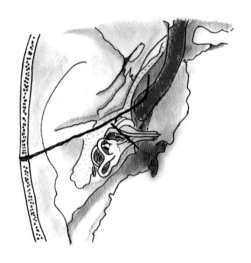

**Figure 7.1**

Diagrammatic representation of longitudinal and transverse fractures of the temporal bone

appearance of discoloration of the skin over the mastoid (Battle's sign).

Patients with temporal bone fractures may develop ear bleed and occasionally CSF otorrhea with deafness, which may be conductive or sensorineural. These fractures may give rise to vertigo and facial paralysis, which, however, are commonly seen with transverse fractures.

In a case of vehicular accident or trauma to the head, these fractures often appear in combination with other skull fractures or brain injuries (contrecoup injuries), which may be associated with air in the cranium. In these cases, interdisciplinary co-operation with the neurosurgeon is required. Today, high resolution computed tomography of the temporal bone makes it possible to define priorities in the treatment of these patients.

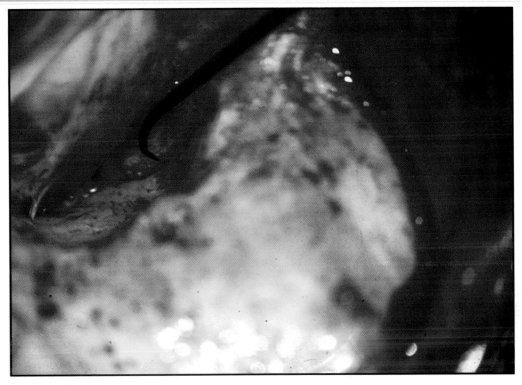

**Figure 7.2**

Intraoperative photograph of longitudinal fracture of the temporal bone involving the external auditory canal and going towards the second genu of the facial nerve

## Pathology

### Longitudinal Fractures

Eighty percent of temporal bone fractures are longitudinal (Figs 7.2 and 7.3) and usually result from blows to the temporal or parietal areas (Proctor, Gurdjian and Webster, 1956). The fracture line usually runs anterior to the otic capsule and involves the external and middle ears resulting in bleeding from the ear with conductive hearing loss due to ossicular disruption. Since the fracture does not involve the otic capsule, sensorineural hearing loss is not seen. The facial nerve canal is usually spared and facial palsy occurring in longitudinal fractures is usually delayed in onset and is due to nerve edema in most of the cases (Figs 7.4 a and b). Such cases can be conserved and medical line of management, which includes steroids, will result in improvement of the function of the facial nerve. Facial nerve exploration should be undertaken in well-selected cases only.

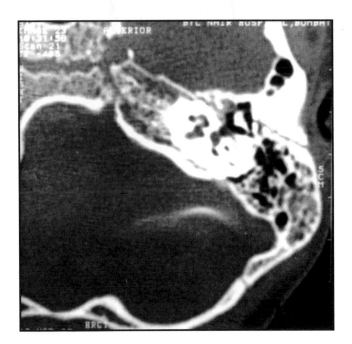

**Figure 7.3**

CT scan axial view showing a longitudinal fracture of the temporal bone

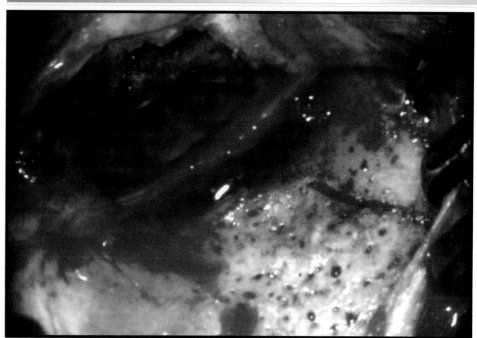

Figure 7.4 a

Intraoperative photograph showing fracture of the mastoid cortex, on exploration, it was involving the dura but there was no CSF leak

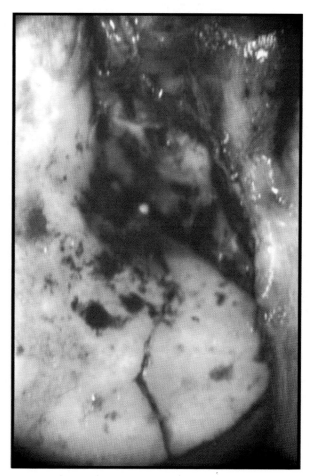

Figure 7.4 b

Intraoperative photograph showing fracture of the mastoid cortex and the posterior bony wall of the external auditory canal

## Transverse Fractures (Fig. 7.5)

Transverse fractures usually result from frontal or occipital blows and account for approximately 20% of temporal bone fractures (Proctor, Gurdjian and Webster, 1956). The fracture line passes through the otic capsule thus damaging the inner ear. A pure transverse fracture can result in a hemotympanum and since the tympanic membrane is usually intact, it is not associated with bleeding from the ear. It is characterized by sensorineural hearing loss, tinnitus, nausea, vomiting, vertigo and facial palsy on the affected side. However, in an unconscious patient with head injury, these signs may be missed until recovery occurs. Fifty percent of these patients develop facial nerve palsy, which is immediate in onset.

## Mixed Fractures (Figs 7.6 and 7.7)

In severe head injuries there may be a combination of the longitudinal and transverse fracture with a loose fragment of bone, which can result in facial palsy if it lies over the facial nerve. The facial palsy seen in these mixed (comminuted) fractures of the temporal bone

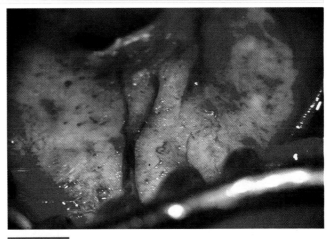

**Figure 7.6**

Intraoperative photograph showing comminuted fracture of the temporal bone. One of the fragments of the fracture was pressing over the mastoid segment of the facial nerve

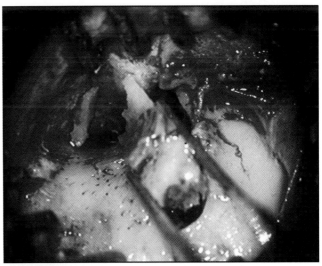

**Figure 7.7**

Intraoperative photograph showing removal of a loose fractured segment of the mastoid bone in a case of temporal bone fracture of the same patient (Fig. 7.6) during facial nerve decompression

is usually immediate in onset. Also, the head injury resulting in such a massive complex fracture of the temporal bone is usually severe and associated with brain edema or pneumocranium and prolonged unconsciousness as well as other skull bone fractures with CSF leakage. Depending on the type of trauma there may be fractures of other bones like those of the extremities.

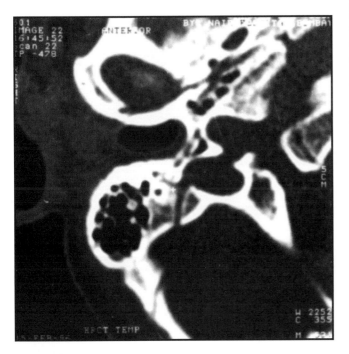

**Figure 7.5**

CT scan axial view showing transverse fracture of the temporal bone

53

## Clinical Features

1. Deafness—Conductive or sensorineural or mixed.
2. Hemotympanum and bleeding from ear, which may become purulent at a later date. The bleeding from the ear may also be due to the laceration of the skin from the external auditory canal.
3. Facial palsy—Lower motor neuron type. It may be immediate or delayed in onset.
4. Vertigo—Severe initially but usually tends to subside on its own within two to three weeks. This is usually due to hemorrhagic labyrinthitis or leakage of the perilymphatic fluid through the fracture line.
5. Lateral rectus palsy—This is usually on the side opposite to the fracture and is due to intraorbital hematoma secondary to contrecoup brain injury (Figs 7.8 a to d).
6. CSF otorrhea and otorhinorrhea—This is rarely seen and may occur in severe head injury resulting in fractures of skull bones other than the temporal bone. In the presence of an intact tympanic membrane CSF may leak through the nose going via the eustachian tube.
7. Discoloration of the skin over the mastoid—Battle's sign.
8. Presence of other injuries to the skull may manifest themselves as unconsciousness, neurological deficit and bleeding from various sites.
9. CT scan will show evidence and type of fracture as well as associated fractures of other skull bones, hematoma, brain edema and pneumocranium (Figs 7.9 a and b, Fig. 7.10).

## Management

The priority in management of a patient of head injury with fracture temporal bone depends on the general condition of the patient. Unconsciousness and vital parameters are stabilized first.

Investigations required should be done on emergency basis. For the diagnosis of fractures of the

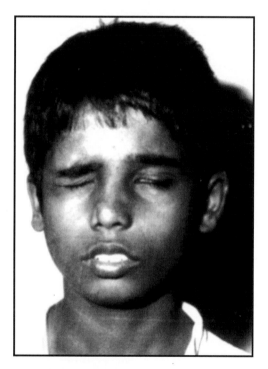 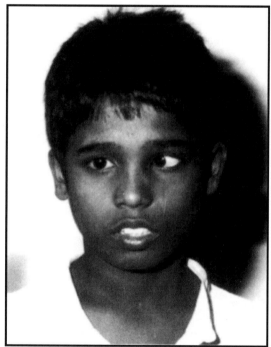

**Figures 7.8 a and b**

Clinical photograph of a patient with left side facial palsy and right sided lateral rectus palsy due to vehicular accident causing fracture of the left temporal bone and hematoma in the right orbital cavity

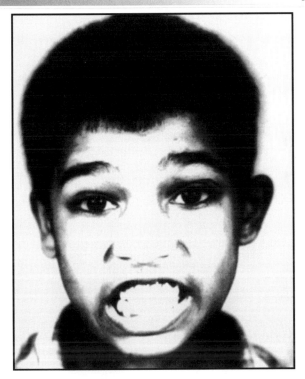
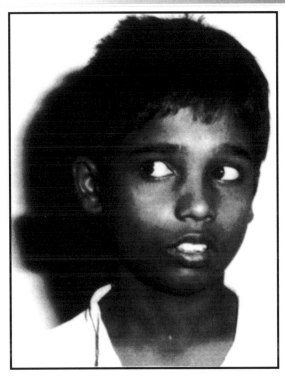

**Figures 7.8 c and d**

Postoperative photograph of the same patient (Figs 7.8 a and b) three months after decompression of the facial nerve. Note the improvement in facial function and recovery of lateral rectus palsy

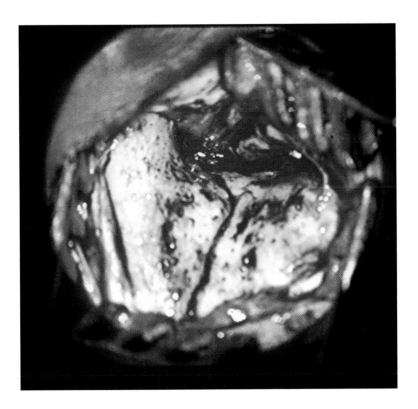

**Figure 7.9 a**

Intraoperative photograph showing an extensive longitudinal fracture of the right temporal bone involving the second genu anteriorly and the posterior cranial fossa posteriorly

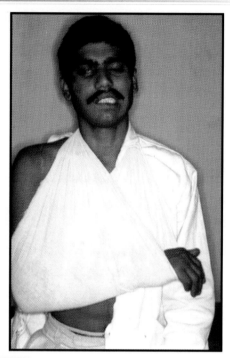

**Figure 7.9 b**

Clinical photograph of the same patient (Fig. 7.9a) with right facial palsy and upper limb fracture

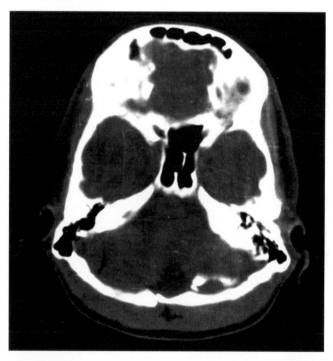

**Figure 7.10**

CT scan axial view showing longitudinal fracture of the temporal bone with fractures of other cranial bones. Patient also had a fracture of the shaft of femur

temporal bone, High resolution computed tomography (HRCT) of the temporal bone is the investigation of choice. Previously, X-rays of the mastoid like the Stenver's, Owen's and Schüller's views were done. However, they are very poor diagnostic indicators of temporal bone fractures.

Once the patient is stable the conductive hearing loss and facial palsy are to be treated. Vertigo usually subsides within 2-3 weeks and the sensorineural hearing loss is irreversible. Vertigo is either due to labyrinthine concussion or due to perilymph leakage. If it is due to concussion and edema, it tends to resolve with medical management. Whereas in case of a perilymph leakage, the vertigo subsides due to complete leakage of the middle ear fluid resulting in a dead ear followed by compensation.

In a case of conductive hearing loss, repair of the torn tympanic membrane and disrupted ossicular chain is performed.

Unusually, we have observed that in cases of facial palsy related to fractures of the temporal bone that present late, the facial nerve sheath may be caught between the fractured fragments and the fracture heals. This results in bands that are formed in the nerve sheath which compress the nerve. These bands have to be cut during the procedure of facial nerve decompression to relieve the nerve of its strangulating effects, thus improving the chances of a functional recovery (Figs 7.11 a and b, Fig. 7.12).

In the case of facial palsy a decompression of the facial nerve is performed in its entire length after the hematoma is evacuated from the mastoid antrum. If the fracture has involved the posterior meatal wall and there is associated anteriorly placed facial nerve, decompression may be performed by the canal wall down technique. We prefer to decompress the nerve in all its segments (labyrinthine, tympanic and mastoid) and then if required lift it out of its canal followed by widening of the fallopian canal and replacement of the nerve back in the widened canal (Grewal et al 1998) (Figs 7.13 and 7.14). The exploration of the facial nerve should be preferably performed within 72 hours as after 72 hours the process of Wallerian degeneration sets in. According to McCabe (1972), if 72 hours have passed, the optimum time for the repair

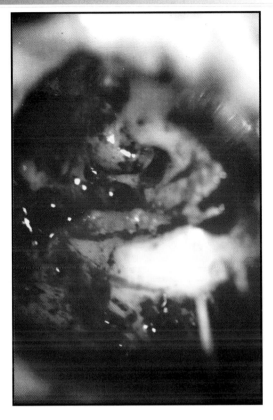

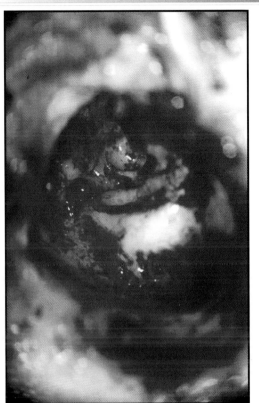

**Figure 7.11 a**

Intraoperative photograph of facial nerve decompression done in a case of long-standing facial palsy due to fracture temporal bone. There was no indication of the fracture line (probably healed as it was long-standing). The nerve sheath shows bands compressing the nerve leading to the nerve herniating in between

**Figure 7.11 b**

Intraoperative photograph of the same patient (Fig. 7.11a) during facial nerve decompression. The compressing bands were cut and the nerve relieved of its strangulating effect

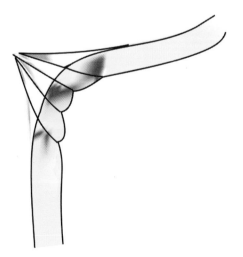

**Figure 7.12**

Diagrammatic representation of the nerve sheath causing strangulation and herniation of the nerve when pulled by the fracture line

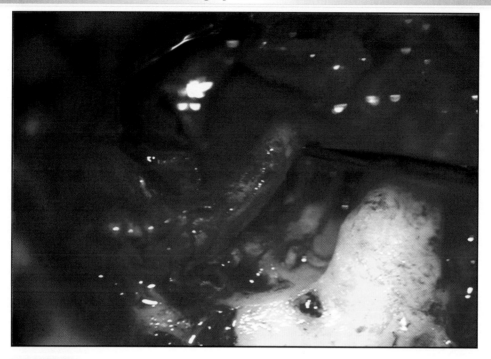

**Figure 7.13**

A case of longitudinal fracture of the temporal bone in which the facial nerve was decompressed and taken out of the fallopian canal (High Power). The canal was widened and nerve was replaced back

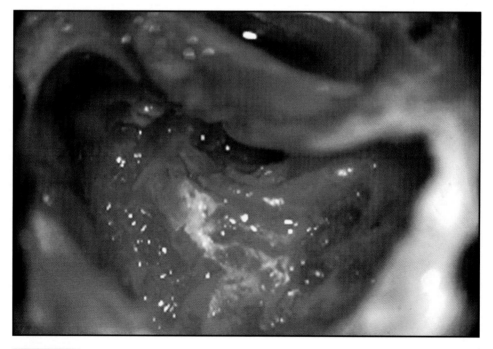

**Figure 7.14**

Intraoperative photograph showing facial nerve decompressed in a case of fracture of the temporal bone. The fracture line was involving the fallopian canal leading to facial palsy

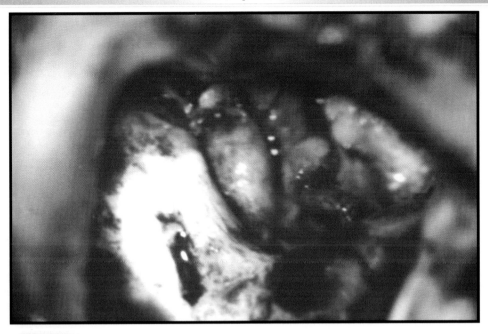

**Figure 7.15**

Intraoperative photograph of the facial nerve where the nerve sheath is slit open and a markedly edematous nerve is observed. The patient had a fracture of the temporal bone, which resulted in facial palsy along with sudden hearing loss and giddiness. The patient presented late and on exploration the incus was compressing the facial nerve with edema of the nerve. The ossicle was removed and the nerve sheath was slit. The patient also had a lateral semicircular canal fistula

of the facial nerve is on the 21st day as the nerve cell body is maximally capable of passing the axoplasmic filaments across the neuronal gap. If decompression is carried out, we advocate not to perform any ossiculoplasty since if the ossicle/prosthesis slips, it can damage the bare nerve (Fig. 7.15). Rarely, a combined management involving a neurosurgeon and ENT surgeon is required in extensive fractures.

## BIBLIOGRAPHY

1. Grewal DS, Hathiram BT, Manjrekar T, Tankwal P, Patankar MA, Ranawat J: Fractures of the temporal bone. Indian Journal of Otology 1998;4:109-14.
2. Hough JVD, Stuart WD: Middle ear injuries in skull trauma. Laryngoscope 1968;78:899-937.
3. Kettel K: Peripheral facial palsy in fractures of the temporal bone. Archives of Otolaryngology 1950;57:25.
4. McCabe BF: Injuries to the facial nerve. Laryngoscope 1972;82:1891-96.
5. Proctor B, Gurdjian ES, Webstar JE: The ear in head trauma. Laryngoscope 1956;66:16-59.

❈ ❈ ❈ ❈

# CHAPTER 8
# Iatrogenic Injury of the Facial Nerve during Surgery of CSOM

## INTRODUCTION

An injury to the facial nerve represents the otologic surgeons' greatest fear. Surgeons are aware of not only the cosmetic and functional consequences of such a complication, but also related medicolegal aspects. Unfortunately, the fear of damage to the facial nerve may lead to avoidance of the nerve instead of positive identification. The best method of preventing iatrogenic injury to the facial nerve is to identify the nerve and use it as a landmark for finding other structures. When the surgeon can see the full course of the nerve in the operative field he or she will not injure it (Shambaugh and Glasscock, 1990).

Although the normal anatomy of the facial nerve is familiar to most otolaryngologists, the anatomy may be distorted by prior surgery, granulation tissue (which may be tuberculous) or cholesteatoma. In rare instances, the facial nerve may follow an anomalous course, rendering the usual surgical landmarks unreliable (Mayer et al 1976). These circumstances challenge the most experienced otologic surgeon. In the days of the mallet and the chisel, and mastoidectomies without microscope, the incidence of iatrogenic facial injuries was high. Now, the use of micromotors, irrigation, suction and the operating microscope with an improved anesthetic technique has greatly reduced this complication of ear surgery (Grewal and Hathiram 1999).

However, facial palsy still does occur due to some or the other reason such as:

1. Destruction or distortion of landmarks for identification of the facial nerve.
2. Anomalous course of the facial nerve.
3. Anomaly of the facial nerve.
4. Faulty operative technique-drilling and handling of sharp instruments.

5. Slipping of material used for reconstruction such as prosthesis, bone or cartilage.

Injury during otologic surgery is most likely to occur in the second genu and the tympanic segment (Green et al 1994). The surgical landmarks for the tympanic segment include the cochleariform process, the oval window and the pyramidal process. The lateral semicircular canal and the cog are the landmarks while approaching the facial nerve (tympanic segment) through the mastoid. Landmarks for the mastoid segment include the lateral semicircular canal, the fossa incudis and the digastric ridge. The posterior semicircular canal may be a useful landmark in the well-pneumatised temporal bone (Green et al 1994).

In cases of intact canal wall mastoidectomies and ossiculoplasties, the facial nerve may be damaged by:

1. Inadvertent handling of incus which can injure the dehiscent second genu of the facial nerve.
2. Graft materials and prosthetic materials like PORP, TORP and synthetic materials kept for ossicular reconstruction might injure the dehiscent horizontal facial nerve and second genu.
3. While widening the aditus from the antrum, dehiscent second genu can be injured.
4. When antrum is exposed through Macewan's triangle, if the dural plate is low lying and the antrum is small and contracted, the surgeon may drill more anteriorly and inferiorly and can injure the nerve in the mastoid segment. This was the most important etiologic factor in our experience (Fig. 8.1).
5. While performing a posterior tympanotomy, it may be preferable to identify the facial nerve first and then to do a posterior tympanotomy otherwise the mastoid segment of facial nerve can be injured.

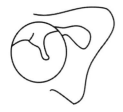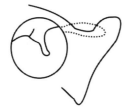

**Figure 8.1**

Diagrammatic representation of the normal mastoid antrum and a narrow contracted and posteriorly placed mastoid antrum with a low lying dura which predisposes to facial nerve injury

In case of canal wall down mastoidectomies, the most common site injured was the second genu (Grewal 1996).

1. Second genu can be injured while operating in the floor of the fossa incudis and on removal of posterior buttress.
2. Mastoid segment can be injured while lowering the facial ridge especially when the nerve is dehiscent, malformed or its course is anomalous.
3. In children, postauricular incision itself can cause facial palsy if it is extended inferiorly because of the absence of a well formed mastoid tip.

## Tests for Facial Nerve Function

1. A detailed history and facial nerve examination is essential. Important points in the history include
   i. Onset of palsy
      • Time of onset.
      • Completeness of the palsy at the onset.
   ii. Duration of palsy.
   iii. Progress of palsy.
2. Schirmer's test and test for taste sensation of anterior 2/3rd of the tongue can be of value if properly performed, to identify the probable site of injury.
3. Electrodiagnostic tests are more reliable if available. Nerve conduction study helps to detect the type of injury and also helps in evaluating the postoperative conduction through the repaired nerve segment/graft. Electromyography helps in prognosis.

## Management of Iatrogenic Facial Palsy

Iatrogenic injury of the facial nerve represents a special problem, especially when there is an unexpected post-operative facial palsy.

After surgical exploration of the facial nerve further management depends upon:
   i. Site of injury.
   ii. Extent of nerve section—partial or complete.
   iii. Cut nerve ends are in approximation or there is a loss of nerve segment.
   iv. Whether cut ends are fibrotic or not.
   v. The time interval between onset of palsy and time of exploration.

It is imperative to ascertain whether the palsy is complete or incomplete and whether the nerve was identified by the surgeon during the surgery. If there is partial recovery after six hours of surgery, medical line of management is followed. However, if after six hours of surgery, there is no recovery or the palsy continues to worsen, early surgical exploration is merited. If the injured nerve is identified intraoperatively during surgery by the operating surgeon, the repair is carried out at the same time.

On early surgical exploration there may be either a cut injury or some compressing factors, which may be the cause of the facial palsy. If there are compressing factors present such as ossicle/cartilage/bone wax, they should be removed and the facial nerve decompressed (Figs 8.2 to 8.7). If there is a cut injury, it should be repaired by suturing and/or nerve grafting (See flow chart).

## Methods to Restore Functional Continuity of the Facial Nerve

1. If the nerve is intact but edematous and congested, decompression of the nerve has to be done till healthy nerve is found on either side. The nerve decompression should be done by removing the fallopian canal all around with widening of the canal using diamond burrs. Slitting of the nerve sheath should be done only to drain a suspected intraneural haematoma.
2. If there is a partial cut to the nerve early nerve suturing with 8-0 nylon/prolene gives best results.

61

**Flow Chart 8.1**

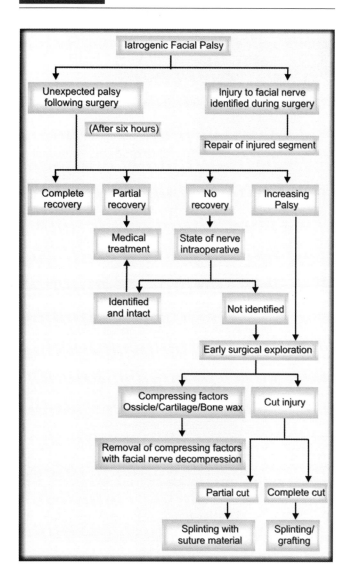

technique is natural self-adhesiveness without use of sutures. If the nerve graft is placed in the facial canal, sutures may not be necessary; but if fallopian canal is destroyed by excessive drilling then connective tissue should be placed underneath the graft and sutures should be taken. It is better to take only one suture with 8-0 nylon/prolene at each end. It is more important to keep upper end of anastomotic site more stable because axonal nerve regeneration is from above downwards. It is also important to remove approximately 1mm of neurilemmal sheath at the anastomotic ends and to bevel the cut ends. The ideal time of nerve grafting is within 30 days of onset of palsy but it can be done as a reinnervation procedure up to 18 months following injury.

5. If there is complete transection with the upper stump not being available for reinnervation and the duration of palsy is more than 18 months, the procedure of choice is facio-hypoglossal anastomosis. But this procedure has the disadvantage of mass movement, lack of emotion, and paralysis of tongue muscles which may be over come by the facio-hypoglossal "jump" anastomosis technique.

6. The main factors that influence the results following the nerve repair are the technical flaws that might down-grade recovery; these include:
   i. Lack of suitable nerve ends
   ii. Tension at the suture line
   iii. Infection

Regeneration of an uninterrupted nerve occurs approximately at the rate of 1 mm per day. The first sign of returning of function is the improvement in tone of the paralyzed muscles. Other techniques of facial re-animation include :
a. Sling operations using tendon or fascia.
b. Free neurovascular repair.
c. Muscle transposition—masseter or temporalis.

Protection of eye—mainly to prevent exposure keratitis includes:
a. Wearing dark goggles.
b. Tarsorrhaphy.

3. If there is complete transection of the nerve and length of nerve damaged is less than 5 mm re-routing and providing end to end anastomosis gives the best results. Although, in our experience, we did not perform re-routing.

4. If there is complete transection and both cut ends are apart, not in approximation even after re-routing, nerve grafting preferably with greater auricular nerve gives the best results. It is preferable to take the nerve graft a little longer than the defect and the preferred anastomotic

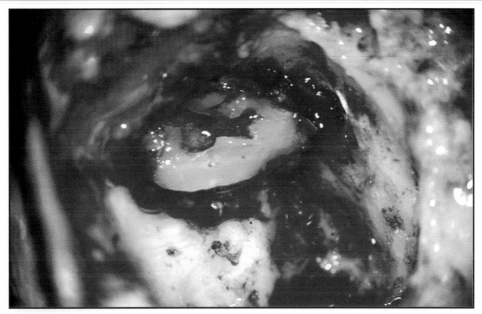

**Figure 8.2 a**

This patient underwent ear surgery when the surgeon had to abandon the operation as there was massive bleeding from a high jugular bulb. The tear in the jugular bulb was sealed by bone wax. Postoperatively there was complete facial palsy. The mastoid was explored at a later date and bone wax was removed

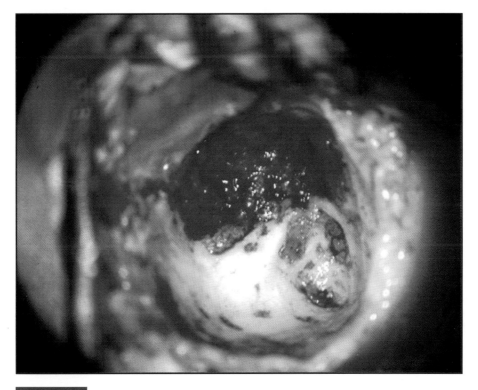

**Figure 8.2 b**

On removal of bone wax, there was an anteriorly placed facial nerve running over the promontory

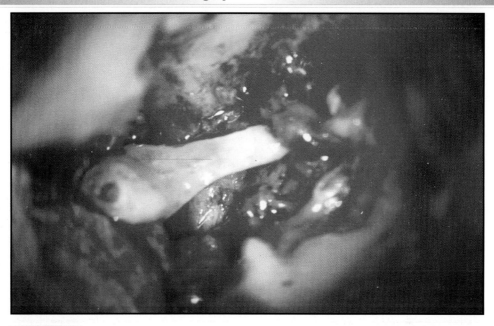

**Figure 8.3 a**

Intraoperative photograph showing injury to the dehiscent facial nerve in its tympanic segment due to the displaced refashioned incus used for reconstruction of the ossicular chain (seen on 10th postoperative day). Note the shallow socket which resulted in the ossicle graft slipping from the stapes head

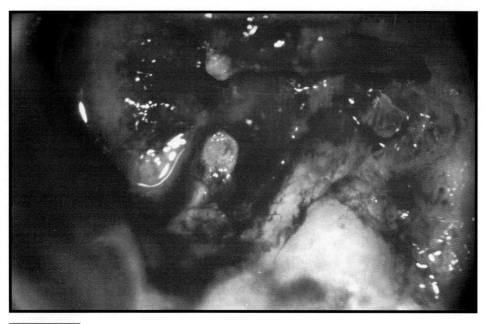

**Figure 8.3 b**

Note the lesion over the dehiscent facial nerve after removal of the displaced incus resulting in neuropraxia

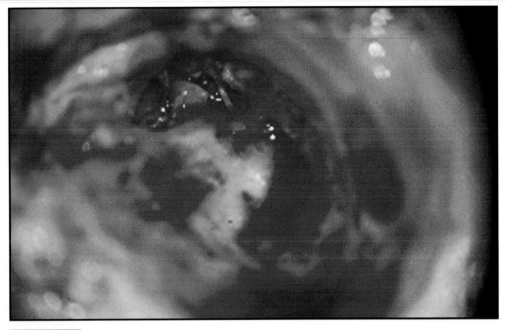

**Figure 8.4 a**

Intraoperative photograph showing the displaced(tilted) incus used for reconstruction of the ossicular chain resulting in injury to the dehiscent facial nerve in its tympanic segment

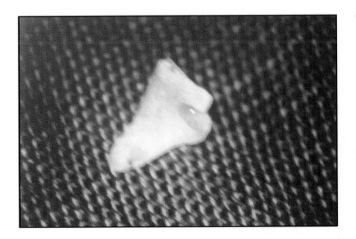

**Figure 8.4 b**

Note the deep socket which is improperly fashioned on the incus which resulted in an unstable assembly with the stapes head resulting in tilting of the ossicle

c. Gold weight for upper eyelid.
d. Eyelid spring.
e. Lower eyelid tightening with temporalis muscle transfer.

## Type of Nerve Injuries

The facial nerve may be injured during surgery either by a sharp instrument or by a cutting burr. When a sharp instrument injures, it usually leads to a cut injury of the nerve, which may be partial or complete. A partial cut usually results in palsy of the angle of the mouth and spares the eye (due to the representation of fibres in the nerve) whereas, a total cut injury results in complete palsy involving the hemiface. However, we have seen that a partial cut injury, at times may present as a complete palsy especially when the patient comes late (after few months) and this fact is explained by us on the basis of our intraoperative finding of a granuloma which is seen to completely encircle the injured nerve segment. This in our view, results in compressing the whole thickness of the nerve and a complete palsy occurs inspite of only a partial cut injury being present. Recovery is rapid once the granuloma is peeled off and nerve ends are approximated.

When the nerve is injured by a cutting burr, the damage depends on the surface of the burr, which comes in contact with the nerve:

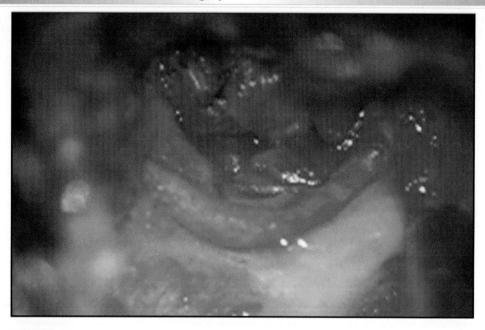

**Figure 8.5**

Intraoperative photograph of revision tympanomastoidectomy for facial palsy following type III tympanoplasty using incus showing a decompressed facial nerve in its tympanic and mastoid course. Note that the nerve is edematous, congested and running over the stapes foot plate. Also note the deep indentation at the site of trauma by the incus, where it pierced the nerve running over the stapes footplate

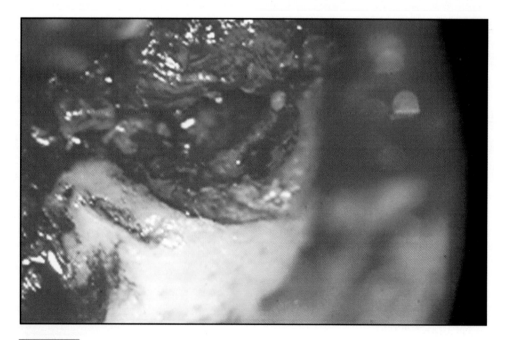

**Figure 8.6**

Injury to the dehiscent facial nerve in its mastoid segment due to the jagged edges of a cartilage graft used to reconstruct the tympanic membrane during myringoplasty

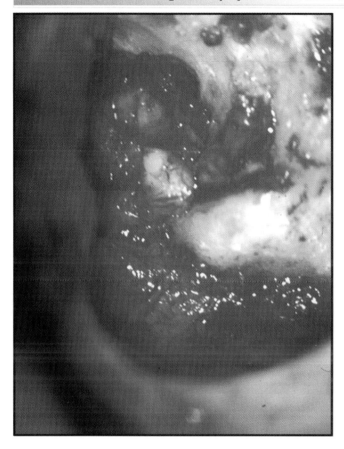

**Figure 8.7 a**

Cartilage used for ossiculoplasty causing facial nerve palsy in a patient. On exploration, the cartilage was seen directly over a dehiscent facial nerve causing compression

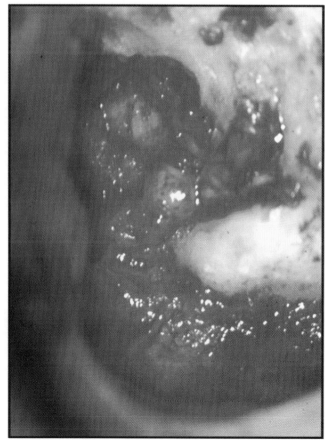

**Figure 8.7 b**

Note the edematous injured facial nerve after removal of the cartilage

a. If the tip of the burr comes in contact with the nerve, the injury ranges from abrasion to transection of the nerve with a segment of nerve missing.

b. If the side of the cutting burr comes in contact with the nerve, it can lead to injury ranging from superficial abrasion to loss of a large segment of the nerve as the nerve is wrapped around the burr and torn out of its canal due to the impact of the rotating burr (Figs 8.8 to 8.12).

### Technique of Nerve Repair

Suturing of the cut ends when there is no loss of facial nerve segment is not always possible as infection and granulation result in bleeding which makes identification of the cut ends difficult since the ends are also edematous, congested and friable. This also makes tying of a knot difficult since the sutures cut through the nerve ends. Also if a knot (of prolene or nylon) is tied we have observed that the cut ends tend to get inverted thus impeding physiological nerve reunion and the knot being big as well as non-absorbable can result in pressure and neuropraxia once the graft is in place. Due to these reasons, we have only passed an 8-0 nylon/prolene suture material through the cut ends of the nerve without tying a knot. The nylon/prolene is passed approximately 2 mm on either sides of the cut ends and the ends are approximated gently by sliding over the nylon in a manner similar to sliding of

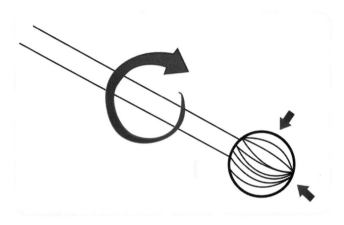

**Figure 8.8**

Diagrammatic representation of a cutting burr. Note the tip and the side of the burr, which can cause different types of injuries to the facial nerve

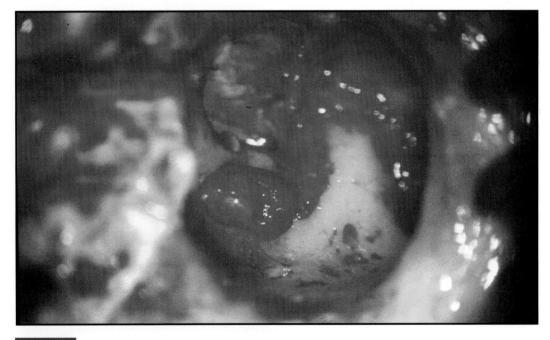

**Figure 8.9**

Intraoperative photograph of a cut injury of the facial nerve (sickle knife)

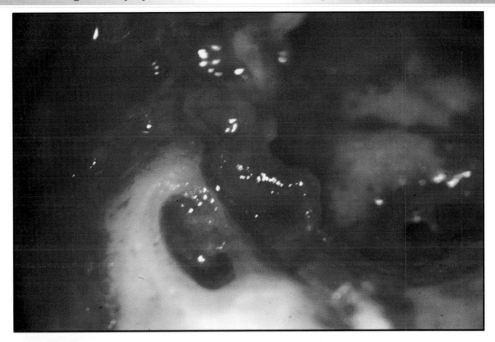

**Figure 8.10 a**

Note the iatrogenic injury to the facial nerve as well as the lateral semicircular canal resulting in a facial palsy and labyrinthine fistula with the membranous labyrinth clearly seen through the fistula

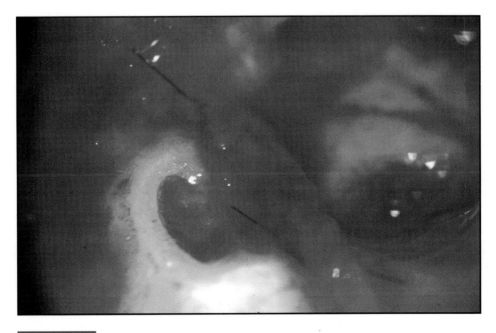

**Figure 8.10 b**

Repair of the facial nerve at two sites using 8-0 prolene and closure of the fistula using a temporalis fascia graft

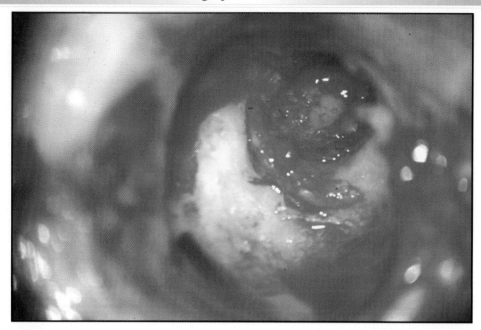

**Figure 8.11 a**

Intraoperative photograph showing herniation of the facial nerve through its sheath at the second genu

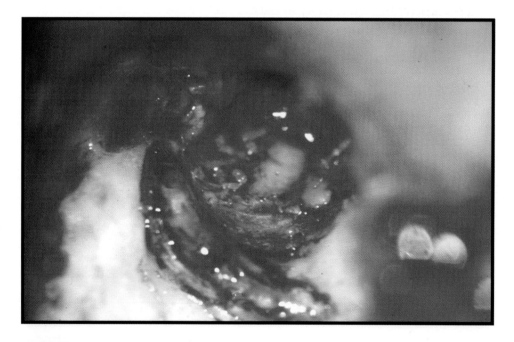

**Figure 8.11 b**

The facial nerve sheath was slit open to reveal a partial cut injury to the facial nerve which was repaired

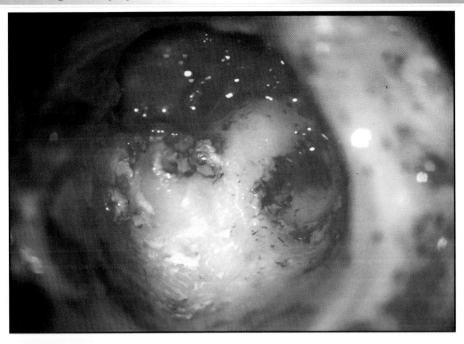

**Figure 8.12 a**

This patient had immediate facial palsy following tympano- mastoidectomy. On exploration, a low lying dura and cut ends of the facial nerve due to faulty and excessive drilling are seen

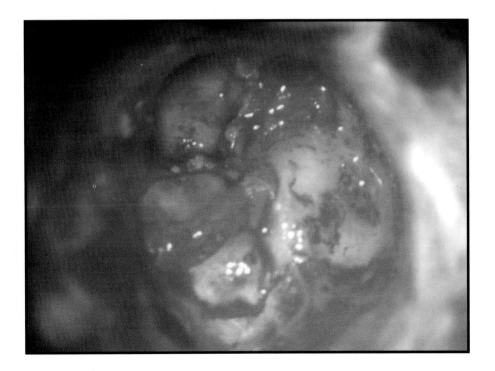

**Figure 8.12 b**

Cable grafting by using greater auricular nerve

curtains over a rod. This helps to approximate the ends without damage to the nerve tissue. The ends of the suture material are tagged under the nerve sheath, which is reposited back over the nerve, thus helping the suture material to remain in place. This is then covered and supported by a temporalis fascia graft (Grewal and Hathiram 1999).

In our opinion this technique works on the following principle:

a. The suture material serves as a splint, keeping both nerve ends stable and in approximation, which aids in nerve healing and reunion.

b. This technique can be compared to a creeper, which requires the support of a stick to grow in a particular direction. Similarly, the suture material merely serves as a scaffolding for guiding the cut ends of the nerve to unite in the correct and desired direction for recovery of nerve function (Figs 8.13 to 8.16).

## Location of Site of Nerve Injury

In a revision mastoid surgery, all the landmarks are destroyed and the usual warning signs indicating that the nerve is being approached such as decrease in size of mastoid air cells, bone becoming whiter and denser and the bleeding from the perineural vessels, are absent. Also there is granulation tissue due to faulty

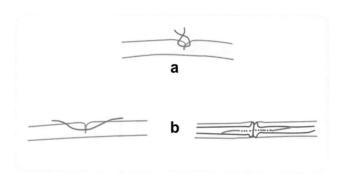

**Figure 8.13**

Diagrammatic representation of (a) the inversion of the cut ends of the nerve after tying a knot and (b) the maintenance of the nerve ends in anatomical approximation when a suture material is passed through the cut ends without tying a knot therefore acting as a splint. Subsequently nerve sheath is placed over the suture ends

mastoid surgery, which bleeds during revision surgery.

Therefore, in our experience during previous surgery the nerve was always exposed and then injured. Now on opening the mastoid and clearing the granulations we see a red inflamed site along the course of the facial nerve, which is the site of injury. We initially identify this "red spot" and proceed to decompress the nerve on either side of this trauma. We use this sign for identification of site of injury since it is most consistent in the absence of usual anatomical landmarks and easy to detect once the eye is trained to look for it.

## Prevention of Iatrogenic Injury

Facial nerve trauma can be avoided by (Grewal 1996):

i. Making the surgeon competent to identify the nerve in its anatomical and anomalous course.

ii. To identify important landmarks during surgery.

### Making the Surgeon Competent

a. Temporal bone dissection—This helps in knowing the exact course, size, shape, and appearance of facial nerve under microscope.

b. To watch visual aids preferably videos—to know and learn the exact method of handling facial nerve during surgery, its variations and pathological conditions leading to its palsy. Also videos can be seen repeatedly and at leisure. Various surgical conditions can be reviewed within a specific time period.

c. To see facial nerve surgery intraoperatively so as to become familiar with depth perception, instrumentation, operative set-up and management of patient and surgical expertise.

### To Identify Important Landmarks

Tympanic part does not as such require any landmarks as it is seen easily. But it can still be located by noting the stapes and processes cochleariformis and above it the nerve continues upto the cog as the labyrinthine segment.

In the mastoid segment and second genu, the pyramidal process, lateral semicircular canal, short process of incus and the diagastric ridge give the exact

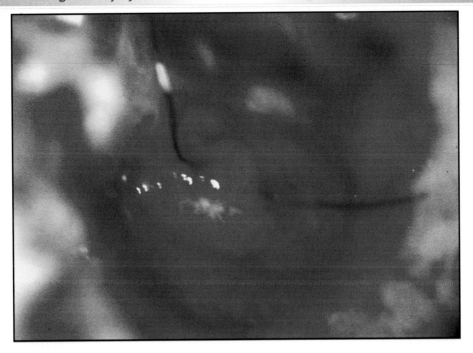

**Figure 8.14**

Intraoperative photograph of a suture material in position holding the cut ends stable and in approximation acting as a splint. Note the absence of the knot

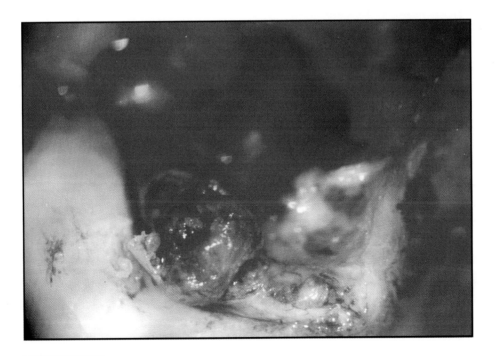

**Figure 8.15 a**

Long standing cut injury to the facial nerve showing formation of a granuloma

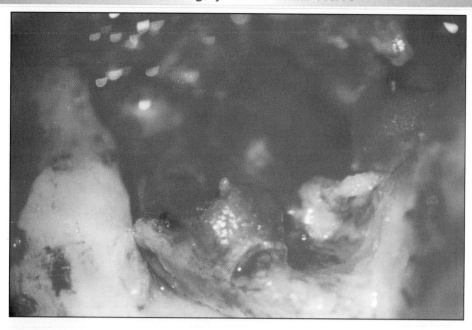

**Figure 8.15 b**

The cut edges were refashioned and sutured

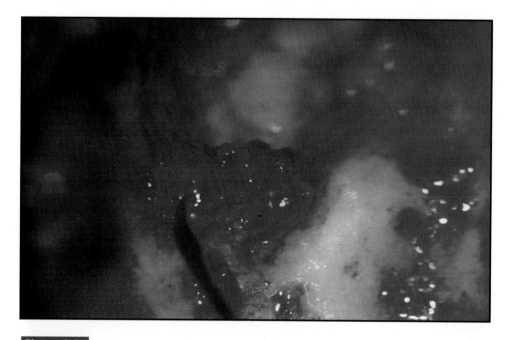

**Figure 8.16**

Intraoperative photograph of a decompressed facial nerve. The sickle is pointing towards the granuloma formed following previous surgery

level of the facial nerve. While performing mastoid exenteration the warning signals, which indicate that the facial nerve is being approached, are:

a. Mastoid cells become smaller.
b. Bone becomes whiter and denser.
c. Bleeding from vessels over the nerve sheath.

However, one has to realize that in case of an iatrogenic palsy, all anatomical landmarks are destroyed and hence the above mentioned indications/warning signals are usually absent. Hence, the surgeon has to largely depend on his surgical expertise and experience.

## CONCLUSION

The facial nerve being the longest and thickest structure to run through the mastoid and middle ear should be easily identified as a thick white cord. Avoidance of iatrogenic trauma to the facial nerve mainly includes the surgeon's thorough knowledge and familiarity with the normal anatomical landmarks, anomalous course of the facial nerve and the skill in handling the nerve when required to do a timely exploration and to decompress or repair the damaged facial nerve. Even after surgery, medical line of treatment is important which includes steroids, antibiotics and physiotherapy under supervision.

In our experience, nerve conduction studies and EMG are important prognostic investigations and help to detect the stability, presence and conductivity of the graft or the sutured nerve ends. Hence, we perform these tests at regular intervals to monitor the response of impulses being conducted through the repaired nerve.

## BIBLIOGRAPHY

1. Green ID Jr, Shelton C, Brackman DE: "Iatrogenic facial nerve injury during otologic surgery" Laryngoscope 1944;104:922-26.

2. Green ID Jr, Shelton C, Brackman DE: "Surgical management of iatrogenic facial nerve injuries" Otolaryngology and Head and Neck Surgery 1994;111:606-10.

3. Grewal DS, Hathiram BT: "Facial nerve repair after iatrogenic injury following tympanomastoidectomy surgery—Our technique" Indian Journal of Otology 1999;5:131-33.

4. Grewal DS: "Iatrogenic facial palsy following surgery of chronic suppurative otitis media" Indian Journal of Otology 1996;2:161-65.

5. Mayer TG, Crabtree JA: Archives of Otolaryngology 1976;102:744-46.

6. Shambaugh, Glasscock: Surgery of the Ear, 4th ed: Facial nerve Surgery, W.B.Saunders and Co 1990;435-65.

❋ ❋ ❋ ❋

# CHAPTER 9
# Facial Nerve in the Parotid Gland

## Surgical Anatomy of the Parotid Gland

The parotid gland is a unilobular, flat and triangularly shaped salivary gland, lying mainly in the retromandibular sulcus. It is enclosed within a fibrous capsule, which sends septae into the glandular substance dividing it into lobes.

The facial nerve emerges from the stylomastoid foramen (3-4 mm deep to the outer edge of the bony EAC), runs anteriorly, inferiorly and laterally to enter the posteromedial aspect of the parotid gland. The nerve bisects it unequally into a large part, which lies lateral to the nerve, called the superficial lobe and a smaller part, which lies medial to it, called the deep lobe. Most parotid tumors are found superficial to the facial nerve since they affect the superficial lobe. In between the two lobes is the faciovenous plane (of Patey) containing the facial nerve along with the retromandibular vein and the branches of the external carotid artery.

## Landmarks of the Facial Nerve in Parotid

Different methods to locate the nerve in the parotid gland are:

i. Tragal pointer (of Conley):   The nerve is located medial and about 1 cm inferior to the tragal cartilage.
ii. Tympanomastoid suture:   This is located at the apex of the vaginomastoid angle or valley of the nerve. It is the angle where the vaginal process of the tympanic portion of the temporal bone meets the mastoid process. The facial nerve runs just deep to this suture.
iii. Styloid process:   The nerve passes lateral to the styloid process at the skull base.
iv. By tracing the terminal branches of the facial nerve backwards:

- The ramus frontalis is located by a line from the tragus to lateral canthus.
- The ramus buccalis is located by a line from the tragus towards the alae of the nose parallel to the zygoma but 1 cm below.
- Ramus mandibularis is near the angle of the mandible at a point 4-4.5 cm from the attachment of the lobule of the pinna.

v. Tendon of the posterior belly of digastric muscle.
vi. Posterior auricular vein or the retromandibular vein.

## Facial Nerve Division and Branches in the Parotid and Face

The nerve divides into two main divisions one cm beyond its entry into the parotid gland at the Pes anserinus.

1. Upper division is stouter and consists of the temporal, zygomatic and upper and lower buccal branches.
2. Lower division is thinner and consists of mandibular and cervical branches. Sometimes the buccal branch may arise from the bifurcation.

Lower zygomatic branch lies just superior to the parotid duct. Damage to the mandibular branch results in paralysis of depressor anguli oris during surgery of the upper neck such as parotidectomy, submandibular gland excision, etc (Figs 9.1a and b and 9.2).

## Involvement of the Facial Nerve in Relation to Parotid

The facial nerve may be damaged in the following lesions involving the parotid gland:

1. Congenital lesions.
2. Inflammatory lesions.

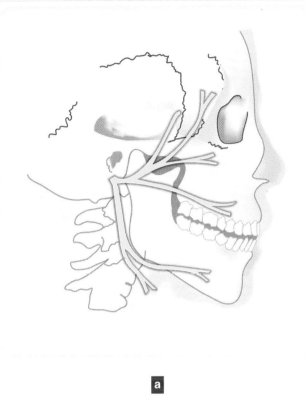

a

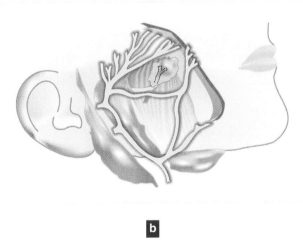

b

**Figures 9.1 a and b**

Diagrammatic representation of the various branches of the facial nerve in parotid gland

3. Traumatic, which may be iatrogenic or accidental trauma.
4. Neoplastic lesions.

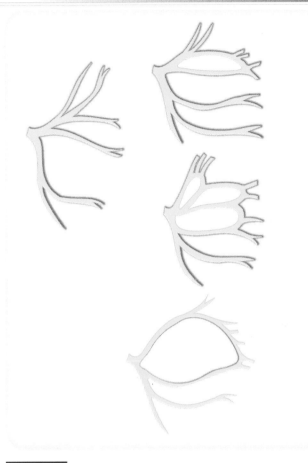

**Figure 9.2**

Diagrammatic representation of the common variations of facial nerve branching in the face

### Facial Nerve Injury due to Trauma

Penetrating trauma, lacerations and injury to the facial nerve are the commonest causes of extratemporal facial nerve paralysis.

Facial nerve injuries are classified as:
1. Compression
2. Pulsion—Pulling/tearing of the nerve as in severe injury to the nerve during birth
3. Crushing
4. Transection—Clear-cut injury with or without missing segment

### Facial Nerve in Parotid Neoplasms

1. Lymphangiomas of the parotid gland surround the facial nerve and then spread downwards into the submandibular gland.

2. Facial nerve should be dissected out from beyond the periphery of the neoplasm.

3. Pleomorphic adenomas may lie in intimate contact with the undersurface of facial nerve or may involve the facial nerve sheath.

### Trauma to the Facial Nerve during Surgery

1. Part of the parotid, which lies superficial to the facial nerve, is peeled off the nerve together with the tumor in partial parotidectomy.

2. In total conservative parotidectomy, the nerve may be injured when the tumor is being delivered through a gap between the branches of the facial nerve or being scooped out inferiorly from under the facial nerve.

### Facial Nerve Weakness after Parotidectomy

It is usually temporary and commonly affects the mandibular and frontal branches of the facial nerve. It is more prone to occur in elderly patients, in those with slender rather than stout branches where an unusual degree of trauma occurs in the vicinity of nerve, due to pressure or traction on the nerve or constant suction on its surface. It may also occur due to excessive drying of its sheath or heat from diathermy.

### Facial Nerve in Malignancy of the Parotid

Adequate resection of tumor is performed and the branches or even the main trunk of facial nerve may be resected, if involved.

Facial nerve involvement (extratemporal) in congenital lesions is seen in the following conditions:
1. Malformations of ear.
2. Excessive growth of styloid process which leads to hypoplasia of the nerve.

### Injury to Facial Nerve in Parotid (Fig. 9.3)

Facial nerve divisions in parotid have various connections and form a webbed network called Pes anserinus.

Injury to the main trunk or temporozygomatic or cervicofacial divisions is always repaired.

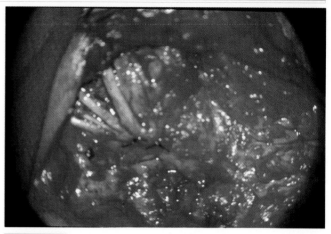

**Figure 9.3**

Intraoperative photograph showing sutured branches of the facial nerve in the parotid following cut injury due to a stab wound

In clear facial lacerations, with immediate onset facial nerve palsy, repair is undertaken spontaneously in the first 3 days, or if not possible, then 3 weeks later.

In case of gross contamination, proximal and distal segments should be identified and tagged.

Primary end-to-end anastomosis results in greater functional return than interposition grafting with multiple anastomoses.

In gunshot wounds or blasts, extensive soft tissue injury occurs and if nerve loss is extensive then interposition graft is used.

In parotid surgery when facial nerve is to be preserved, it is stimulated near the stylomastoid foramen before wound closure if there is no movement then careful inspection under microscope is carried out for evidence of injury like accidental ligature on nerve or crush injury.

When facial nerve injury occurs posterior to the anterior margin of masseter muscle concomitant injury to parotid duct is looked for.

### BIBLIOGRAPHY

1. Johns M, Kaplan M: Neoplasms-Salivary Glands. Cummings C. W. 2:1039-41.

2. May M: Disorders of facial nerve, Scott-Brown's Otolaryngology, 6th ed, 3:24/10-12.

3. Miehlke J: Parotid tumors & Facial nerve. Surgery of facial nerve 125-28.

4. Proctor B: Anatomy of the facial nerve. Otolaryngologic Clinics of North America 1991;24(3):499-503.

5. Shaheen OH: Benign salivary tumours. Scott-Brown's Otolaryngology, 6th ed, 6:352-55.

6. Warren AJ, Osguthorpe D: Management of trauma of the facial nerve: Otolaryngologic Clinics of North America, 1991;24(3):587-92.

❋ ❋ ❋ ❋

# CHAPTER 10
# Hemifacial Spasms

Hemifacial spasm is the symptom complex of unilateral facial nerve hyperactive dysfunction characterized by the onset of mild and intermittent spasms in the orbicularis oculi muscle that gradually progress in severity and frequency. It spreads gradually to include all the muscles of facial expression. A mild muscular weakness may also be seen over a period of months or years (Janetta et al 1977).

The facial spasms may be primary or secondary. Primary spasms are the idiopathic hemifacial spasms while secondary spasms are usually secondary to a recovering facial paralysis and are often combined with contractures. It may be occasionally confused with a facial tic. However, a facial tic is psychogenic. It is the habit of shutting the eyelids or blinking, distorting the mouth and wrinkling the nose. Patients suffering from facial tics usually require psychiatric help.

The idiopathic hemifacial spasms of one side of the face are agitated by paroxysmal, clonic, voluntary and episodic muscular contractions. The spasms are more noticeable in the lower eyelid and the oral commissure. This unpleasant grimace is aggravated under emotional tension, which makes the patient irritable especially in the presence of a third person.

## ETIOLOGY

The etiology of idiopathic hemifacial spasms is unknown. There are several theories proposed to explain it:

a. *Otologic theory:* In this the causative lesion is an edema of the facial nerve or a fibrous constriction of its sheath (Woltman et al, 1951; Pulec, 1972). Those who accepted this etiological thesis postulated the existence of an irritable focus in any segment of the facial nerve, which causes a short-circuiting of impulses.

b. *Neurosurgical theory:* The lesion could be caused by a continuous and prolonged pressure upon the seventh nerve by a vascular structure in the posterior cranial fossa (Janetta, 1972).

c. *Neurological theory:* The pathological condition could be located in the motor nucleus of the facial nerve in the brainstem (Wartenberg, 1952; Crue et al, 1968). Supporters of this theory believe that these impulses originate in the ganglion cells of the facial nerve in brainstem.

The lack of a consensus on the causes of idiopathic hemifacial spasms suggests that the exact cause is still not known and in different cases, it may have different etiologies. Clinically, it is very difficult but not impossible to determine in a patient with this disease, whether the lesion is in the nucleus, the cerebello-pontine angle or in the fallopian canal.

## TREATMENT

Generally, medical measures fail to control the symptom and surgery is the only available therapeutic or palliative option. Operative treatment depends largely on the various etiological theories. The medical line of treatment includes drug treatment and also treatment with botulinum toxin.

### Drug Treatment

Various drugs have been tried for the treatment of hemifacial spasms. They reduce the severity and the frequency of spasms but the results are disappointing. Carbamazepine may be used in doses from 100 mg once daily to 12 hourly to a maximum of 200-400 mg given 8 hourly. The drug dosage is increased over a period of 2-3 weeks to get an optimum therapeutic concentration of 30-50 µmol/lt and to prevent sedative side effects. Phenytoin may be used in a range of 150-500 mg (average 300 mg) depending upon the tolerance of the patient; to achieve a plasma level of about 40-80 µmol/lt. Clonazepam 0.5-2.0 mg 8 hourly is effective at times (Cull and Will, 1995).

## Botulinum Toxin Injection

Injection of Botulinum toxin type A is another effective method of temporary relief from hemifacial spasms. Botulinum toxin is produced by the bacteria Clostridium botulinum. It has a molecular weight of 150kDa and is capable of neuromuscular blockage due to its single polypeptide chain to dichain molecules held by disulphide bonds. The heavy chain portion of the molecules binds irreversibly to the presynaptic cholinergic nerve terminals at specific receptor sites causing a reversible neuromuscular junction blockade. It has shown good results in 90% of the patients treated for hemifacial spasms.

0.1 to 0.2 ml of a diluted form of toxin may be injected around the eye in the orbicularis oculi muscle and in the zygomaticus major muscle for periorbital and perioral twitches (Fig. 10.1). The effects of the toxin become apparent within 2-7 days and maximum effects are seen by the 10th day. The effects of the treatment last for about 10 weeks.

The disadvantages include:
1. Local pain at the injection site
2. Periorbital bruising
3. Diplopia
4. Ptosis
5. Ectropion with misting of vision
6. Drooping of the angle of the mouth.

## Operative Procedures

The procedures to relieve the spasms can be divided into a number of categories based on the theoretical factors implicated.

### *Facial Nerve Needling*

This treatment is based on the theory originally proposed by Fergusson (1978) that the deafferentiation of the central pontine nucleus secondary to peripheral nerve injury results in abnormal discharges that are manifested as hemifacial spasms. McCabe and Boles (1972) and Karnik and Jain (1973) have proposed that the motor fibres that supply the facial musculature originate in the suppressor area of the motor cortex and any damage to this leads to the overactivity of the facial nerve causing hemifacial spasms.

Facial nerve needling cuts down peripheral motor units and causes muscle weakness. However, it gives relief from the spasms. The sites include the mastoid segment (Celis et al, 1974), the stylomastoid foramen (Wakasugi, 1972) or the branches within the parotid gland (Fisch and Esslen, 1972). Ludman and Choa (1985) in their study of 62 patients have described the operation of transtympanic facial nerve needling. Out of the 54 patients that followed up 22 patients showed complete or almost complete relief of spasm in the first operation itself. A few of the patients had to undergo the operation again. Ogale et al (1995) in their study of 10 patients who underwent transtympanic facial nerve needling in the horizontal segment have reported 6 patients to be completely relieved of their symptoms.

The operative procedure for transtympanic facial nerve needling entails an endomeatal approach with

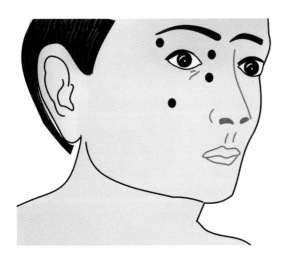

**Figure 10.1**

Diagrammatic representation showing sites of injection to treat periorbital and perioral twitching

exposure of the tympanic segment of the facial nerve. The fallopian canal of the facial nerve is thinned and removed. The facial nerve is then punctured with a fine microsurgical pick making 4 to 6 punctures. This technique was based on cutting down the number of motor units in the peripheral musculature by inducing lesions in the peripheral course of the facial nerve. Here minimal facial weakness is traded for relief of spasms.

The advantage of transtympanic facial nerve needling is the ease of the procedure but the chances of recurrence are higher than with microsurgical decompression technique.

### Partial Neurectomy

This treatment is based on the same principle as facial nerve needling. Hemisection of the facial nerve can be done in the mastoid segment (Ludman and Choa, 1985) or longitudinally splitting at the cerebello-pontine angle (Fan, 1993). Of the 33 cases Fan (1993) treated, none of the 20 cases that followed up for 1 year showed recurrence. The failure rate in this series was 10%.

### Vascular Decompression of Facial Nerve

This treatment is based on the belief that this disorder is peripheral in origin due to decompression of the nerve trunk. The compression of the nerve could be due to an aberrant blood vessel loop at the Root Exit Zone (REZ) at the cerebello-pontine angle or the porous of the internal auditory meatus (Gardner and Sava 1962, Janetta et al 1977).

Janetta et al (1977) in their study of forty-five patients with classical hemifacial spasms have described the decompression of the facial nerve at the cerebello-pontine angle. The cause of hemifacial spasm was found to be a vascular cross-compression usually by an arterial loop. The facial root exit zone is decompressed by changing the axis of the arterial loop through interposition of a small prosthesis of a non-reabsorbable spongy material, e.g. a piece of muscle or a Ivalon sponge or Teflon between the artery and the facial nerve and the vestibulocochlear nerve. The artery may be large such as a vertebral or the basilar

artery or small such as the postero-inferior cerebellar artery or the antero-inferior cerebellar artery. They have reported excellent results in 38 of the 45 patients on which the surgery was performed.

Any posterior fossa neurosurgical operation, no matter how skillfully performed, is more hazardous than an operation in which the nerve is approached extracranially, with the risk of cochlear nerve damage, aseptic meningitis, or a small chance of mortality. Nowadays, with the use of an endoscope for this procedure, the morbidity and the complication rate have significantly decreased.

### Other Procedures

Some of the other procedures that can be done for hemifacial spasms include:
• Facio-hypoglossal anastomosis (Andrew 1981).
• Total decompression of the intratemporal course of the facial nerve (Pulec 1972)
• Orbicularis oculi stripping (Elston 1988).

However, the results have not been very encouraging.

## BIBLIOGRAPHY

1. Andrew J: Surgery for Involuntary Movements. British Journal of Hospital Medicine 1981;26:552-28.
2. Blaubach AC, Castillo AH: Idiopathic Hemifacial Spasm—New Method of Surgical Treatment. Acta Otolaryngologica 1974;77:221-27.
3. Crue BL, Todd EM, Carregal EJ: Compression of Intracranial portion of the facial nerve and section of nervus intermedius for hemifacial spasm. Bull Los Angeles Neurology Soc 33:70.
4. Cull RE, Will RG: Diseases of the nervous system. Davidson's Principles and Practice of Medicine 1995;17:1021-1123.
5. Elston JS: The clinical use of botulinum toxin. Seminars in Ophthalmology III 1988;249-60.
6. Fan Zhong: Intracranial longitudinal splitting of the facial nerve—A new approach for hemifacial spasm. Annals of Otology, Rhinology and Laryngology 1993;102(2):108-09.
7. Ferguson J: Hemifacial spasm and the facial nucleus. Annals of Neurology 1978;4:97.
8. Fisch U, Esslen E: The surgical treatment of hemifacial spasm. Archives of Otolaryngology 1972;95:402-05.
9. Gardner WJ, Sava GA: Hemifacial spasm—A reversible pathophysiologic state. Neurosurgery 1962;19:240.
10. Hawthorne MR, White K: Practical use of botulinum toxin in head and neck dystonia. Recent Advances in Otolaryngology 1995;7:253-70.

11. Janetta PJ, Abbssay A, Maroon JC, Ramos FM, Albin MS: Etiology and definite microsurgical treatment of hemifacial spasm. Journal of Neurosurgery 1977;47:321-28.

12. Karnik PP, Jain JC: Hemifacial spasms. Indian Journal of Otolaryngology 1973;25:31-34.

13. Ludman H, Choa DL: Hemifacial spasm. Operative treatment. Journal of Laryngology and Otology 1985;99:239-45.

14. McCabe BF, Boles R: Surgical treatment of essential blepharospasm. Archives of Otolaryngology 1972;81: 611-18.

15. Ogale SB, Chopra S, Thakkar S: Transtympanic facial nerve needling. Acta Otolaryngologica 1995;115:405-07.

16. Pulec JL: Idiopathic facial spasm- Pathogenesis of segmental decompression. Presented to the American Otological Society on April 24th 1972, Palm beach, Florida.

17. Wakasugi B: Facial nerve block in the treatment of facial spasm. Archives of Otolaryngology 1972;95:356.

18. Wartenberg R: Facial nerve block in the treatment of facial spasm New York: Oxford University press 1952;80.

19. Woltman HW, Williams HL, Lambert EM: An attempt to relieve hemifacial spasm by neurolysis of the facial nerve. A report of two cases of hemifacial spasm with reflections on the nature of the spasm, the contracture and mass movement. Proceedings of Staff Meeting of Mayo Clinis 1951;26:36.

�֎ �֎ ✖ ✖

# CHAPTER 11
# Syndromes Associated with Facial Palsy

## A. MELKERSSON-ROSENTHAL SYNDROME

Melkersson-Rosenthal syndrome is a rare neuromyo-cutaneous disorder characterized by a triad of recurrent facial paralysis, recurrent facial and labial edema (cheilitis granulomatosa) and fissured tongue (lingua plicata). In 1928, Melkersson was the first to describe a symptom complex of facial edema and recurring facial palsy. In 1931, Rosenthal added a fissured tongue or "*Lingua plicata*" to this symptom complex, thus completing the triad of recurrent swelling of the lips or the face, alternating facial nerve palsy and fissured tongue. In the past, Hubschmann (1894) and Rossolimo (1901) had described a similar syndrome of relapsing facial paralyses and facial edema. However, Hubschmann did not document the tongue involvement and Rossolimo included migraine headache. In 1945, Miescher described several patients with "*cheilitis granulomatosa*". However, Dhar and Kanwar (1995) failed to find any granuloma from lip biopsy in 5 out of 6 reported cases (Figs 11.1 and 11.2).

Although the Melkersson-Rosenthal syndrome frequently begins in childhood, it was not reported in pediatric literature until 1962 when Ehmann and Stickl described the syndrome in two children aged 22 months and 8 years respectively. It is more common in females than in males (Mistry et al, 1995). The exact etiology is unknown and theories of the etiology of this syndrome include infection, allergy and hereditary and familial causes (Alexander and James, 1972). Carr (1966) has proposed that Melkersson-Rosenthal syndrome is an autosomal dominant trait, while Lygidakis et al (1979) suggest that "*Melkersson-Rosenthal Syndrome gene*" is situated at 9p11 locus.

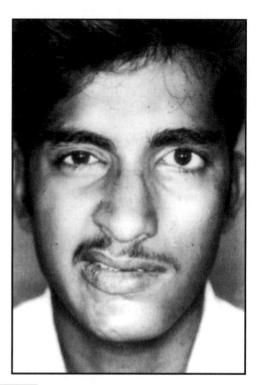

**Figure 11.1**

A patient of Melkersson-Rosenthal syndrome with facial palsy

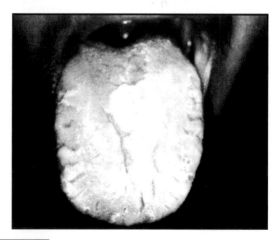

**Figure 11.2**

Fissured tongue in the same patient (Fig. 11.1)

The diagnosis of this syndrome is essentially a clinical one. It can be differentiated from Heerfordt's syndrome by the absence of fever, uveitis and parotitis and it is differentiated from the Aschner's syndrome or "**Double lip syndrome**" by the absence of thyroid enlargement, blepharochalasis and presence of facial palsy (Mistry et al, 1995). It is often associated with migraine, megacolon, facial swelling and stress, which suggest vasomotor instability fundamental to autonomic dysfunction. Rarely other cranial nerves are involved.

However, this syndrome may manifest with two instead of three symptoms (atypical cases) and can, thus, be divided into three clinical forms:

Complete, oligosymptomatic and monosymptomatic The syndrome can occur in the following combinations:

a. Facial paralysis and edema, without lingua plicata.
b. Facial edema and lingua plicata without facial paralysis, or
c. Facial paralysis and lingua plicata without edema (Klaus and Brunsting, 1959).

The facial paralysis is most commonly recurrent, but may be unilateral or bilateral; simultaneous or alternating and occurs only in 1/3rd of the cases (Zimmer et al, 1992). The first episode is commonly seen before the 20th year of life. It is usually complete and of the lower motor neuron type. Facial edema affecting the lips and adjacent areas of the face is the commonest feature. The eyelids, nose, tongue, upper alveolar process and chin may also be affected. Clinically the edema is similar to Quincke's edema. Lingua plicata or fissured tongue is seen in only 25% of cases (Auckland, 1958).

Histological findings of sarcoid-like granulomas from skin or oral mucosa are helpful in the diagnosis. The biopsy of the tongue and the mucosa shows hyperplastic rete pegs, dilated lymphatic channels, fibrosis and perivascular infiltrates of lymphocytes, plasma cells and histiocytes. Granulomatous inflammation is typical of Melkersson-Rosenthal syndrome, but is not mandatory as Melkersson-Rosenthal syndrome is essentially a clinical diagnosis and not a histopathological one.

Therapy for this syndrome is mainly directed to the treatment of facial palsy and correction of the facial disfigurement due to edema. Initially, facial palsy is managed by warm compresses, analgesics, oral corticosteroids, antibiotic eyedrops and ointment, eye shields and active and passive physiotherapy. The facial palsy usually recovers completely, however recurrences are known to occur. Various therapeutic agents have been tried including vitamin D, antituberculous drugs, penicillin, ultrasound, surgical excision along with plastic reconstruction of the facial edema and facial nerve decompression. However, the results are far from encouraging. Rarely facial nerve decompression can be considered if the symptoms last for a longer duration or if the facial palsy fails to resolve in untreated cases. Facial nerve decompression may be done with the hope of preventing the disfiguring facial synkinesis and increasing facial paresis with each episode. If the lip swelling is cosmetically disfiguring, a plastic surgical repair can be performed, whereas the lingua plicata does not merit any therapy.

Recent advances in management include the use of oral clofazimine or laser beam acupuncture according to traditional Chinese medicine that have proved to be helpful in recovery (Hornstein, 1997; Dhar and Kanwar, 1995).

## BIBLIOGRAPHY

1. Alexander RW, James RB: Melkersson-Rosenthal syndrome- Review of literature and report of a case. Journal of Otolaryngology 1972;30:599-604.
2. Auckland G: Melkersson's syndrome. British Journal of Dermatology 1958;70:458-59.
3. Carr RD: Is Melkersson-Rosenthal syndrome hereditary?. Achives of Dermatology 1966;93:426-27.
4. Dhar S, Kanwar AJ: Melkersson-Rosenthal syndrome in India: Experience with six cases. Journal of Dermatology 1995;22:129-33.
5. Ehmann B, Stickl H: Recurring facial paralysis and swelling— A pediatric contribution to the Melkersson-Rosenthal syndrome. Z. Kinderheilk 1962;110:541-43.
6. Hornstein OP: Melkersson-Rosenthal syndrome—A challenge for dermatologists to participate in the field of oral medicine. Journal of Dermatology 1997;24:281-96.
7. Hubschmann Von P: Ueber recidive und diplegie bie der sogenannten rheumatischen facialislahmung. Zbl Neurochir 1894;13:815.

8. Klaus SN, Brunsting LA: Melkersson-Rosenthal syndrome: Persistent swelling of the face, recurrent facial paralysis and lingua plicata: Report of a case. Mayo Clinic proceedings (1959) 34: 365-70.

9. Lygidakis C, Tsankanis C, Ilias A, Vassilopoulusis D: Melkersson-Rosenthal syndrome in four generations. Clinical Genetics 1979;15:189-92.

10. Melkersson E: Ett fall av recidiverande facialispares i samband med angioneurotisk oedem. Hygiea 1928;20:737-41.

11. Miescher G: Uber essentielle granulomatoze Makrocheilie. Dermatologica 1945;91:57-85.

12. Mistry B, Khan S, Gaikwad N, Chandrakiran, Grewal DS, Hiranandani NL: The Melkersson-Rosenthal syndrome. The Bombay Hospital Journal 1995;37:399-401.

13. Rosenthal C: Klinisch-erbbiologischer Beitrag zur Konstitutionspatiologie. Gemeinsames Auftreten von (rezidivierender familiarer) Facialislahmung, angio-neurotischem Gesichtsodem und Lingua plicata in Arthritismus-Familien. Z Gesamte Neurol Psychiatry 1931;131:475-501.

14. Rossolimo GJ: Recidiverende facialislahmung bei migrane. Zbl Neurochir 1901;20:744.

15. Smeets E, Fryns JP, Van Der Berghe H: Melkersson-Rosenthal syndrome and de novo t (9:21) (p11:p11) translocation. Clinical Genetics 1994;45:323-24.

16. Zimmer WM, Rogers III, RS, Reeve CM, Sheridan PJ: Orofacial manifestations of Melkersson-Rosenthal syndrome. Oral Surgery, Oral Medicine and Oral Pathology 1992;74:610-19.

## B. RAMSAY HUNT SYNDROME

Ramsay Hunt syndrome is also known as herpes zoster oticus or herpes zoster cephalicus. This syndrome is associated with facial palsy, hearing loss, dizziness and herpetic eruptions and is caused by a neurotrophic virus, the herpes zoster virus. Hunt (1907, 1908) first described it as a viral prodrome associated with severe pain in and around the ear and vesicles involving the pinna. In its severe form, it may be associated with vesicles on the tongue and buccal mucosa, lower motor neuron facial palsy, sensorineural hearing loss, disturbance of vestibular function or involvement of several cranial nerves (trigeminal, vestibulocochlear, vagus and glossopharyngeal nerves). It is more commonly seen to affect elderly males.

It is caused by a specific neurotropic virus, but the mode of transmission is yet not well known. However, it causes facial palsy due to a severe lymphocytic infiltration of the geniculate ganglion or the intratemporal segment of the facial nerve.

The characteristics which differentiate Herpes zoster oticus from Bell's palsy include absence of complete recovery in approximately 40% patients and failure of recurrence (Bell's palsy is known to recur in 12% cases). Ramsay in his original description proposed that herpes zoster virus causes affection of the geniculate ganglion resulting in ganglionitis and herpetic eruption of the "geniculate zone". This "zone" is supplied by the sensory portion of the seventh cranial nerve and is situated within the auricle and the external auditory canal (Figs 11.3 a and b).

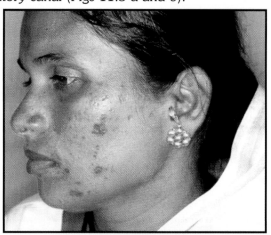

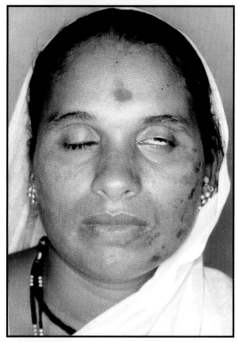

**Figures 11.3 a and b**

A patient of Ramsay Hunt syndrome showing presence of facial palsy and healed vesicles around the pinna

Depending on the clinical presentation, Hunt (1907) classified the Ramsay Hunt syndrome into:
- Herpes auricularis (without neurological signs)
- Herpes auricularis with facial palsy
- Herpes auricularis with facial palsy and auditory symptoms

This classification can also be divided as:
- Herpes auricularis (geniculate herpes)
- Herpes facialias (gasserian herpes)
- Herpes occipitofrontalis (cervical herpes)

Treatment of this syndrome is essentially conservative with the use of:
1. Antiviral agents (Acyclovir): requires a virus specific enzyme for conversion to active metabolite that inhibits DNA synthesis and viral replication.
   *Dose*: 800 mg 5 times/day for 5 days or 5-10 mg/kg/8 hr IV for 7 days
2. Analgesics.
3. Local application of soothing anesthetic ointment.
4. Eye care.
5. Active and passive physiotherapy.

Various researchers like Ballance and Duel (1932), Findlay (1949) and Cawthorne (1965) have advocated facial nerve decompression in cases of Ramsay Hunt syndrome to prevent residual facial palsy and for a speedier recovery. However, the recovery is rarely complete.

## BIBLIOGRAPHY

1. Ballance C, Duel AB: Operative treatment of facial palsy. Archives of Otolaryngology 1932;15:1-70.
2. Cawthorne T: Bell's palsies. Archives of Otolaryngology 1965;81:502.
3. Findlay JP: Herpes zoster of the nervus chorda tympani with facial paralysis. Medical Journal of Australia 1949;2:380.
4. Hunt JR: On herpetic inflammations of the geniculate ganglion—A new syndrome and its complications. Journal of Nervous and Mental Diseases 1907;34:73-96.
5. Hunt JR: A further contribution to herpetic inflammations of the geniculate ganglion. American Journal of Medical Sciences 1908;136:226-41.

## C. MOEBIUS SYNDROME

It is a rare congenital disorder usually characterized by bilateral facial palsy, unilateral or bilateral Abducens palsy, anomalies of the extremities, and involvement of the other cranial nerves especially the hypoglossal with absence of various muscle groups particularly the pectoral group of muscles.

The etiology is unknown but four modes of developmental pathology are known. These are:
1. Hypoplasia or absence of central brain nuclei.
2. Destructive degeneration of central brain nuclei.
3. Peripheral nerve involvement.
4. Myopathies.

Treatment includes reconstructive surgery such as orthognathic and static sling surgery.

## D. HEERFORDT SYNDROME

It is a peculiar symptom complex commonly seen in sarcoidosis. It is also known as uveoparotid fever and is characterized by acute onset uveitis, iritis, parotid enlargement and fever.

This symptom complex is also associated with Bell's palsy and Sjögren's syndrome. The disease is usually benign and resolves without any specific treatment.

## E. FREY'S SYNDROME

### Synonyms
- Auriculotemporal syndrome
- Gustatory hyperhydrosis

### History

Described by Duphenix in 1757.

Lucy Frey, a French neurologist, implicated the auriculotemporal nerve in her account of a Polish cavalry officer with an infected parotid wound.

### Definition

It is a symptom complex that includes localized facial sweating and flushing during mastication of food and cutaneous hyperesthesia in front of and above the ear.

### Etiology

Injury to auriculotemporal nerve gives rise to this syndrome. This nerve can be injured during:

1. Parotidectomy: 35-60% of postparotidectomy patients within 6 weeks to 3 months of operation present with this.
2. Parotid abscess drainage
3. Accidental injury.

### Pathology

The auriculotemporal nerve provides both, parasympathetic innervation to the parotid gland and sympathetic innervation to the sweat glands and subcutaneous blood vessels. The neurotransmitter for both fibres is acetylcholine. Following injury to the auriculotemporal, regrowth of the secretomotor parasympathetic fibres into the distal cut ends of the sympathetic fibres in the skin causes gustatory sweating.

### Treatment

1. Most patients require only reassurance as it resolves spontaneously in a vast majority.
2. Conservative therapy:
   a. Anti-perspirant: Aluminium chloride hexahydrate.
   b. Topical anticholinergics: Glycopyrrolate.
   c. Botulinum toxin A: Interferes with exocytosis of synaptic vesicles at cholinergic nerve endings.
3. Surgical treatment
   a. Tympanic neurectomy: Transection of Jacobsons nerve running on promontory.
   b. Interposition of fascia lata or fat between secretomotor fibres and the skin.
   c. Stellate ganglion block.
   d. Intracranial neurolysis of the glossopharyngeal nerve

To reduce the incidence of Frey's syndrome—modifications of parotidectomy have been developed—elevation of a superficial musculoaponeurotic flap or a sternomastoid flap as interposition to prevent autonomic reinnervation of the skin.

## F. MONDINI'S DEFECT

This is a congenital defect that includes:

1. Cochlea with one and a half turns and the apical coil replaced by a distal sac.
2. Dilated vestibular aqueducts.
3. The organ of corti may be absent or reduced to a mound of undifferentiated cells.
4. The patient is partially or completely deaf.

# CHAPTER 12
# Tumors Causing Facial Palsy

*David Moffat*

## INTRODUCTION

The surgeon with good clinical acumen (Moffat et al, 1998) will be aware of the importance of excluding pathology throughout the whole anatomical length of the facial nerve and its central connections before making a definitive diagnosis of idiopathic facial palsy or Bell's palsy (Fig. 12.1).

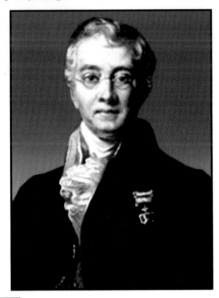

**Figure 12.1**

Sir Charles Bell

Tumors affecting the facial nerve represent one of the greatest challenges facing both the neurotologist and the neuroradiologist. The nerve transgresses the traditional domains of the head and neck surgeon, otologist and neurosurgeon. Mastery of the facial nerve, therefore, represents the cornerstone of the discipline of skull base surgery.

The surgeon depends on accurate imaging by his radiologist at all stages of the management of tumors affecting the facial nerve. Imaging is cardinal in the diagnosis, the determination of treatment and the

follow-up of these patients (Moffat et al, 1993). Furthermore, the role of the interventional radiologist in skull base surgery has become invaluable.

This chapter represents the author's experience of tumors causing facial palsy over a 23-year period in the University Department of Otoneurological and Skull Base Surgery at Addenbrooke's Hospital in Cambridge.

## CLASSIFICATION

Tumors manifesting with facial nerve palsy have been classified into those that are intrinsic to its nerve fibers (Fig. 12.2), and those extrinsic (Fig. 12.3) and adjacent to its course.

The extrinsic tumoral causes arise in the anatomical regions of the:
1. Facial nucleus and supranuclear connections
2. Cerebellopontine angle
3. Temporal bone
4. Parotid

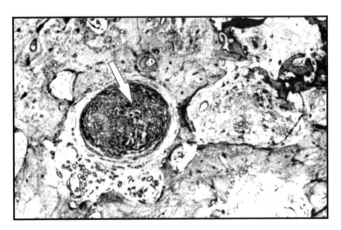

**Figure 12.2**

Histopathology of tumor infiltration of the facial nerve (white arrow)

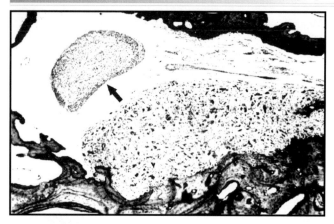

**Figure 12.3**

Histopathology of neoplastic tissue causing facial nerve compression (black arrow)

Tumors of the facial nucleus and supranuclear connections are mentioned for completeness but excluded from review in this chapter.

## Clinical Presentation

A complete facial palsy is easily recognizable (Fig. 12.4) but an early partial palsy is a subtle sign (Figs 12.5 and 12.6) (Moffat, 2001). The earliest sign of a facial palsy is a delay in blinking and the physician should always elicit a blink reflex by asking the patient to look straight ahead and then rapidly tapping the glabellar region with the tester's finger initially hidden from view.

Diagnosis can be a challenge and the symptoms may be slow and insidious (Moffat et al, 1993) and thus the diagnosis may be delayed. The diagnosis of "Bell's palsy" is one of exclusion and a neoplastic cause must be excluded by high resolution imaging of the entire course of the facial nerve.

### *Intrinsic Lesions of the Facial Nerve*

• Schwannoma (neuroma)
• Hemangioma

## Facial Nerve Schwannomas (Neuroma)

Schwannoma is synonymous with neurilemmoma. These tumors arise from the schwann cells of the nerve

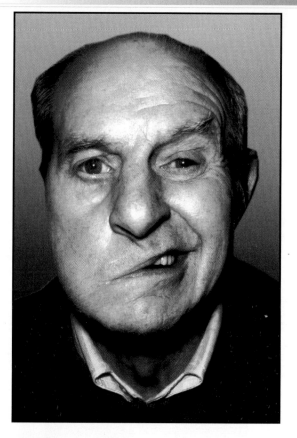

**Figure 12.4**

House Brackmann Grade VI facial palsy

sheath and are often multicentric in origin. They are commonly intratemporal but may occur anywhere along the course of the nerve (Fig. 12.7). The posterior fossa and/or internal auditory canal (IAC) segment is involved in 50% of cases and they comprise 1% of all cerebello-pontine angle (CPA) tumors (Moffat et al, 1993). Eighty percent involve two adjacent segments and are dumb-bell in shape and may have an intratemporal component, normal nerve in the IAC and tumor in the CPA. They may erode the otic capsule. There have been occasional reports of malignancy.

The anatomical location in order of frequency.
• Geniculate ganglion
• Horizontal portion
• Vertical portion
• Internal auditory canal
• Labyrinthine segment
• Extratemporal portion

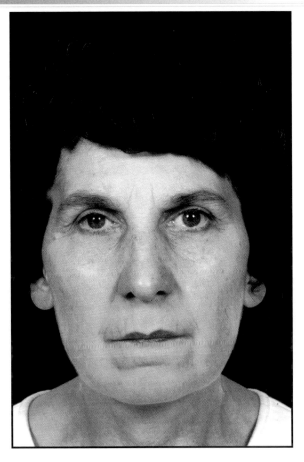

**Figure 12.5**

Normal face at rest

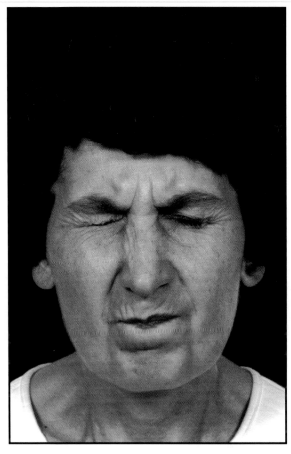

**Figure 12.6**

House Brackmann Grade 2 manifest on screwing up the face

Interestingly only 32% of facial neuromas in the CPA present with facial weakness (Moffat and Ballagh, 1995). Auditory brainstem evoked responses (ABR) are abnormal in 83% of IAC and CPA facial neuromas. Electroneuronography (ENOG) may show a diminished amplitude of the nerve action potential.

Computed tomography (CT) may show a widened fallopian canal (Fig. 12.8) and on both CT and magnetic resonance imaging (MRI) the appearances in the IAC and CPA are identical to acoustic neuroma.

Masses may be present in the posterior and middle cranial fossae. MRI is useful for showing the facial nerve within the temporal bone. T1 weighted images are isointense or hypointense (Fig. 12.9). T2 weighted images are hyperintense and tumors enhance with gadolinium DTPA (Moffat and Ballagh, 1995).

The surgical approach depends on the anatomical location and extent of the tumor. The surgeon should be prepared to operate on the entire length of the facial nerve from the CPA to the parotid. Rerouting of the facial nerve with direct anastomosis is sometimes possible but cable grafting with greater auricular or sural nerve is usually necessary.

## Facial Nerve Hemangioma

These are vascular hamartomas and are predominantly capillary or cavernous (Fig. 12.10). They may present in the temporal bone, IAC or the CPA and may mimic acoustic neuromas (Shaida et al, 2000). They occur most commonly at the geniculate ganglion due to the rich vascular network around it and are usually

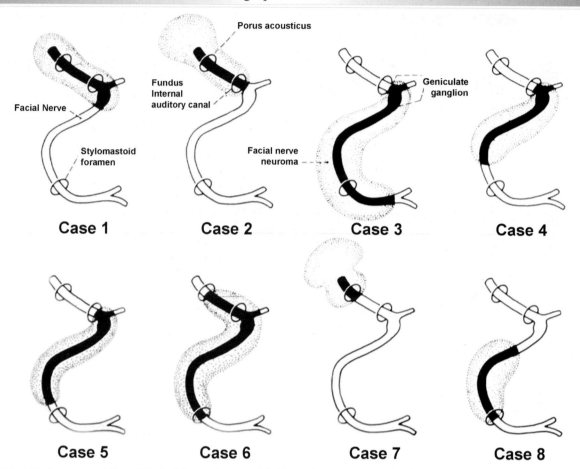

Diagrammatic representation of the facial nerve in cases 1-8. Shaded area represents involvement by facial nerve neuroma.

**Figure 12.7**

Segments of the facial nerve which may be involved in facial neuroma

capillary hemangiomas at this site. Ossifying hemangiomas are due to dystrophic change and bone remodelling.

High resolution CT scanning demonstrates calcium stippling and IV contrast does not enhance the lesion. MRI reveals hyperintensity of the signal on both T1 and T2 weighted images with no contrast enhancement (Fig. 12.11) (Shaida et al, 2000).

They can produce a facial palsy even when very small. Sensorineural hearing loss may occur.

## EXTRINSIC LESIONS OF THE FACIAL NERVE

### Lesions of the Facial Nucleus and Supranuclear Connections

#### Lesions of the CPA

*Vestibular schwannoma*  This is the most common pathology in the CPA occurring in 80.7% of cases (Fig. 12.12) (Moffat et al, 1993). It occurs at a frequency of 1 per 100,000 of the population per year (Moffat

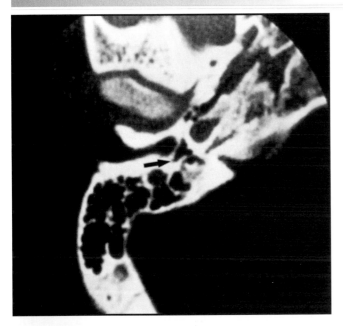

**Figure 12.8**

Axial CT scan of the right temporal bone showing bone erosion in the region of the geniculate ganglion (black arrow)

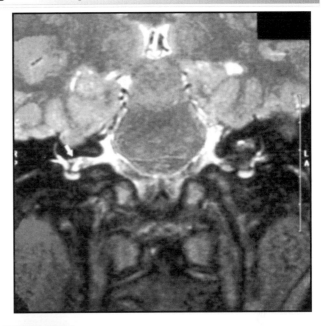

**Figure 12.9**

T2W coronal MRI scan showing a facial neuroma on the right side (white arrow)

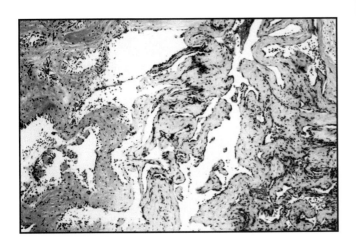

**Figure 12.10**

Histopathological features of a cavernous hemangioma

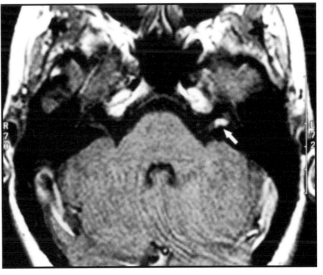

**Figure 12.11**

Axial T1W MRI scan showing the hyperintense lesion in the left IAC without contrast enhancement representing an hemangioma of the facial nerve (white arrow)

et al, 1989). These benign schwannomas grow at a variable rate but in the majority of cases they are slowly growing at a rate of 1-2 mm per year. They may go for long periods without growing. In the Cambridge series of patients undergoing a watch, wait and rescan management policy 60% of tumors were found not to

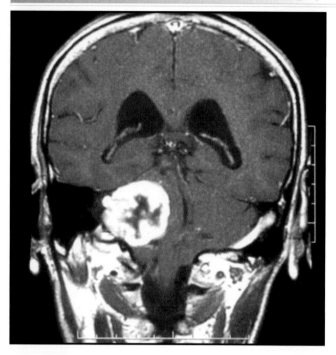

**Figure 12.12**

Coronal T2W MRI scan showing large cystic vestibular schwannoma with marked brainstem compression and shift of the 4th ventricle

be growing over the observation period (Quaranta et al, 2003). For a benign tumor acoustic neuromas bear a remarkably sinister reputation. They are usually silent at first presenting with a little unilateral tinnitus and a progressive sensorineural hearing loss (Baguley et al, 1989). In 10% of cases the deafness is sudden (Moffat et al, 1994) presumably due to compression of the internal auditory artery by the expanding tumor in the IAC. Distortion for hearing more marked than the pure tone threshold would indicate is the hallmark of these tumors. Expansion to touch the trigeminal nerve with its concomitant alteration in sensation on the skin of the face in the distribution of this nerve then occurs and the corneal reflex is depressed. If growth continues, the tumor will begin to indent the brainstem and vestibular disturbance is more likely to occur. Brainstem compression will produce a Brun's nystagmus (Moffat et al, 1988) and increasing unsteadiness on the feet along with obstruction of the cerebrospinal fluid pathways as the tumor completely fills the CPA cistern. Hydrocephalus and raised

intracranial pressure will lead to papilledema and a deterioration in visual acuity. Ataxia and dysdiadochokinesis will result. Neural plasticity particularly in young people will allow remarkable compensation to occur but when decompensation occurs it is often rapid and expedient treatment is needed if the patient is to survive.

CT scanning will only detect vestibular schwannomas when they have grown out into the CPA (Moffat et al, 1993). MRI scanning is the gold standard investigation and often a fast spin echo T2 W image is sufficient to visualize the tumor. If in doubt the patient should be given gadolinium DTPA contrast enhancement.

The management options are:
- Watch, wait and rescan
- Surgery via a translabyrinthine (Hardy et al, 1989. 1, 2), (Moffat et al, 1996), retrosigmoid or middle fossa approach.
- Stereotactic radiotherapy either by single dose or gamma knife therapy or by LINAC in multiple doses.

## RARE TUMORS

Rare tumors of the CPA account for 19.3% of cases (Fig. 12.13). An analysis of the frequency of these rarer

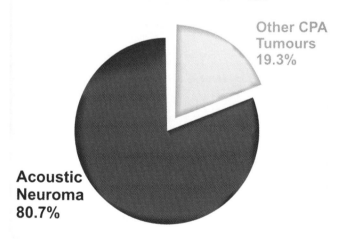

**Figure 12.13**

Exploded pie diagram showing percentage of non-acoustic neuroma lesions of the CPA

lesions can be seen in the pie diagram in Figure 12.14 (Moffat et al, 1993). Meningioma at 6.5% and primary cholesteatoma at 4.3% together make more than half of these rarer CPA tumors.

*Meningioma* Meningiomas account for between 3 and 13% of CPA tumors in the literature and in our series 6.5% (Moffat et al, 1993) (Harada et al, 1994). Ten percent of all meningiomas are in the CPA. Macroscopically they are globular masses with a thin capsule. They displace but do not invade nerves. They arise on the posterior surface of the temporal bone off-centre from the IAC and may be intratemporal.

The characteristic histopathological features can be seen in Figure 12.15.

Clinically patients present with audiovestibular symptoms often of shorter duration than with acoustic neuroma (Baguley et al, 1995). The hearing loss tends to occur later and other cranial nerves are more frequently involved.

Pure tone hearing thresholds tend to be better than in vestibular schwannoma. In 75% of cases the ABR is positive compared with 96% in vestibular schwannoma where a response can be obtained.

In plain X-rays bone destruction or hyperostosis may be seen.

## Unusual Cerebellopontine Angle Tumours

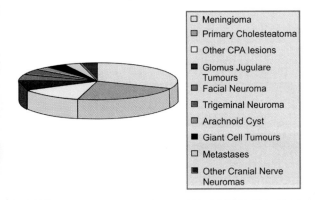

☐ Meningioma
◼ Primary Cholesteatoma
☐ Other CPA lesions
◼ Glomus Jugulare Tumours
◼ Facial Neuroma
◼ Trigeminal Neuroma
◻ Arachnoid Cyst
◼ Giant Cell Tumours
☐ Metastases
◼ Other Cranial Nerve Neuromas

**Figure 12.14**

Pie analysis of rare lesions of the CPA

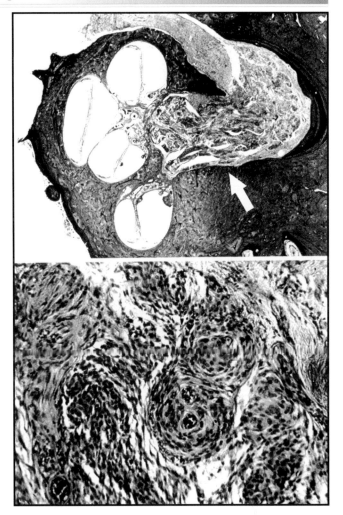

**Figure 12.15**

Histopathology of a meningioma in the IAC (white arrow)

CT scans show the tumor off-centre from the IAC. The tumor mass is dense and homogeneous. There is considerable tumor enhancement with contrast. Calcification and bony changes may be seen.

MRI scans show a tumor which is less intense than a vestibular schwannoma due to their greater vascularity. Delineation between the tumor and the cranial nerves may be seen. The tumors have a flat base since they arise from the posterior face of the temporal bone. They are eccentric to the IAC and the angle between the posterior surface of the temporal bone and a tangent drawn to the tumor is greater than 90 degrees. On the T1 W image the tumor is isointense to hypointense (Fig. 12.16). The T2 W signal is variable

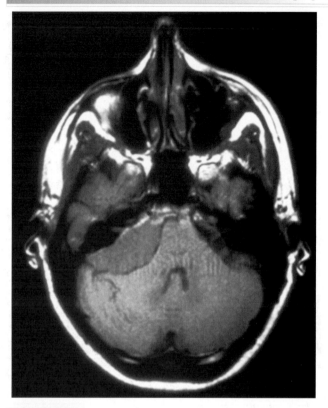

**Figure 12.16**

T1W axial MRI scan of large meningioma arising from the posterior face of the temporal bone. The tumor is hypointense when compared with normal brain tissue. Note the flat base and the tumor mass eccentric to the IAC. The angle between a tangent drawn to the tumor and the posterior face of the temporal bone is more than 120 degrees

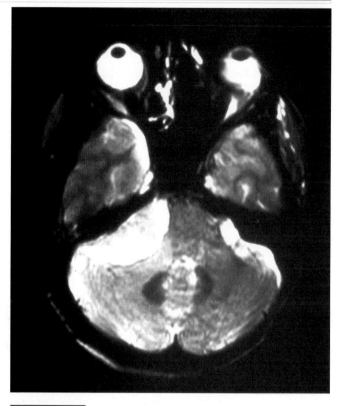

**Figure 12.17**

Same tumor on the T2W image. The tumor is hyperintense

but 50% are hypointense (Fig. 12.17). Gadolinium DTPA enhancement is less than with vestibular schwannoma.

These tumors are not very radiosensitive and surgery is the treatment of choice (Grey et al, 1996) in the fit patient. Recurrences due to incomplete resection are common. Gross and microscopic invasion of the temporal bone occurs frequently and resection of the underlying bone should be undertaken.

*Cholesteatoma (CPA epidermoid)* This pathology comprises 4.3% of CPA tumors. It arises from epithelial rests. The tumor is lined with squamous epithelium and filled with keratin (Fig. 12.18). Cranial nerves are compressed and irritated. The cholesteatoma insinuates between and around nerves rather than displacing them.

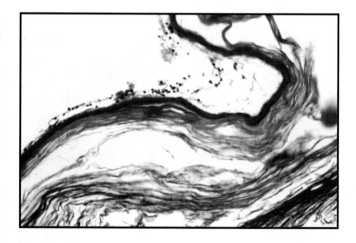

**Figure 12.18**

Typical histopathological appearance of a cholesteatoma with squamous epithelium and layers of keratin

The clinical features include facial twitching which may be an early sign. Progressive facial paralysis is more common than with vestibular schwannoma. Pure tone audiometry often reveals well preserved hearing thresholds (Quaranta et al, 2003) but the speech audiogram tends to reveal poor speech discrimination scores. Dysequilibrium and rotatory vertigo, which may be positional (Beynon et al, 2000), can occur.

Plain X-rays show a smooth scalloped destruction of bone.

CT scanning shows a lesion less dense than brain with irregular margins and eccentric to the IAC. Intravenous contrast shows no enhancement (Moffat et al, 1993).

MRI demonstrates an heterogeneous mass usually hypointense and of the same intensity as cerebrospinal fluid on the T1W image (Fig. 12.19). The T2 W image shows an hyperintense tumor (Fig. 12.20). There is no enhancement with gadolinium DTPA. This com

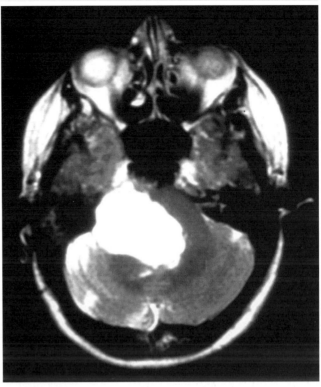

**Figure 12.20**

Axial T2W MRI scan of the same lesion demonstrating the hyperintensity of the mass on the T2

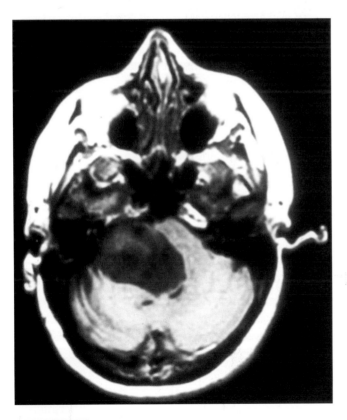

**Figure 12.19**

Axial T1W MRI scan of a CPA cholesteatoma showing an hypointense mass (the same intensity as cerebrospinal fluid)

pares with cholesterol granuloma where the lesion is hyperintense on both the T1W and T2W images (Moffat et al, 1993).

A method of staging CPA cholesteatoma has recently been devised based on the anatomical regions involved (Moffat et al, 2002)

Surgical treatment is hampered by the difficulty in excising the cholesteatoma matrix in its entirety. Denaturing the protein matrix with a defocussed laser may prove to reduce the likelihood of recurrence. The patients require follow-up for life and interval imaging. Recurrences may occur and require further surgery.

*Glomus jugulare tumors (Fisch type D-intracranial)* Fisch type D glomus jugulare tumors account for 1.7% of CPA tumors. The female to male ratio is 2:1 (Moffat et al, 1993).

Classically patients present with pulsatile tinnitus, hearing loss and disequilibrium. Pulsatile headaches may be responsible for a considerable deterioration in the patient's quality of life. Dysphonia, dysphagia and shoulder weakness may be present indicating involvement of the nerves around the jugular foramen, namely the glossopharyngeal, vagus and accessory nerves.

These lesions may be multicentric. Very rarely these tumors are malignant and metastasise (Brewis et al, 2000).

Conductive hearing loss and the otoscopic finding of a red pulsatile mass behind the tympanic membrane arising from the hypotympanum (the rising sun sign) are characteristic features (Fig. 12.21). The jugular foramen syndrome with palsies of all or any combination of the last four cranial nerves may be present. Facial and sixth nerve palsies may also occur.

Pure tone audiometry may be normal but typically there is a conductive hearing loss and bone conduction thresholds may reveal some loss of cochlear reserve in large tumors where there is some erosion of the otic capsule.

CT scanning demonstrates a mass of soft tissue density in the middle ear with erosion of the jugular foramen. There is irregular ragged loss of the margin of the bone of the jugular bulb which may be seen on the axial (Fig. 12.22) and coronal views.

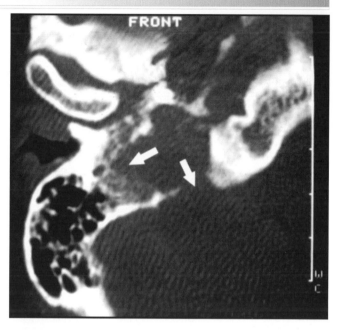

**Figure 12.22**

Axial CT scan of skull base showing ragged erosion of the jugular bulb by a large glomus jugulare tumor (white arrows)

Loss of the bony spur between the jugular and carotid canals is clearly seen on the coronal cuts. Marked contrast enhancement occurs in these tumors.

Multiplanar MRI images give accurate information on the extent of the tumor (Moffat et al, 1993). Marked contrast enhancement occurs with Gadolinium DTPA (Fig. 12.23). It is essential to use CT and MRI in a complimentary fashion in the investigation of glomus jugulare tumors since CT will delineate the extent of the bony erosion and MRI the size and precise anatomical location of the tumor.

MR arteriography may be employed to assess the vascularity and feeding vessels but may not give as much information as conventional carotid ateriography which demonstrates the extent of the tumor and the degree of vascularity. It is important to establish the main feeding vessels not only to assist the surgery but also for preoperative embolization. These tumors have a complex and incredibly rich blood supply which includes feeding vessels from the external and internal carotid arteries and the vertebral artery. The ascending pharyngeal artery is often the main feeding vessel (Figure 12.24) and this may arise from the carotid

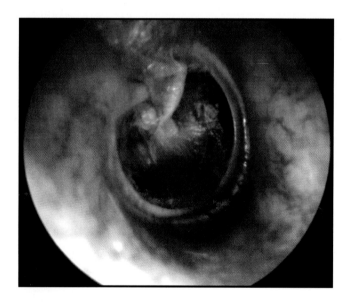

**Figure 12.21**

Otoscopic view of the "rising sun sign" produced by a red vascular pulsatile glomus tumor arising from the hypotympanum

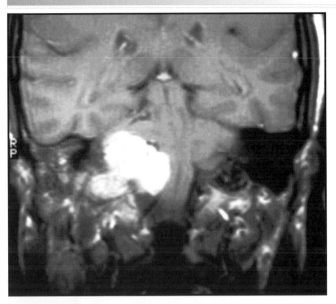

**Figure 12.23**

Coronal T1W MRI scan of vast Fisch type D glomus tumor with marked brainstem compression and shift of the 4th ventricle

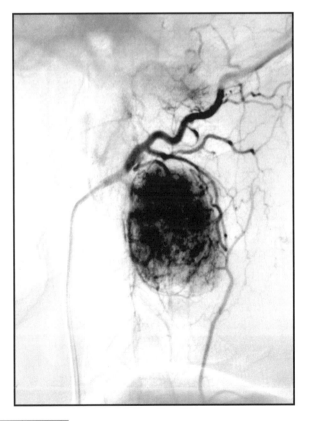

**Figure 12.24**

Carotid arteriogram of a glomus jugulare tumor demonstrating that the ascending pharyngeal artery is the main feeding vessel

bifurcation. The caritico-tympanic arteries are a challenge for the otoneurosurgeon.

These tumors are not very radiosensitive and surgery is the only curative treatment. This is most commonly performed via a trans- and infratemporal approach with blind sac closure of the external auditory canal (Moffat and Hardy1989). The defect is obliterated with fat and fascia lata. Large Fisch type D tumors will require fascial grafting of the dura in the middle and/or posterior cranial fossae. Preoperative selective embolization with coils and feathers is helpful in reducing intraoperative blood loss. Postoperative conformal or stereotactic radiotherapy may be necessary. This can be given as a single dose in gamma knife therapy. New palsies of the IX, X, XI and XII cranial nerves resulting from surgery can pose a real problem particularly for the elderly patient who will not compensate as well as a younger patient. Dysphagia and aspiration may necessitate percutaneous gastrostomy and possibly tracheostomy and medialisation thyroplasty can improve vocal quality. It is therefore important to consider excisional surgery very carefully particularly in the elderly patient with a big tumor who is neurologically intact preoperatively. Removal of the transverse process of the atlas will facilitate access to the jugular foramen and hence increase the likelihood of preserving neural function. Opening the jugular and preserving the wall of the vein and bulb will increase the risk of leaving residual tumor but will decrease the risk of neurological deficit in the last four cranial nerves. Transposing the facial nerve is not always necessary but if it is it will result in a grade II or III face postoperatively.

*Trigeminal neuroma*   These interesting and difficult lesions very rarely cause facial palsy. They present with facial numbness and/or pain and are usually not clinically manifest until they are large.

CT scanning demonstrates smooth enlargement of Meckel's cave or foramen lacerum.

MRI reveals an enhancing iso- or hypointense mass on T1W image (Fig. 12.25). The T2W images are isointense (Moffat et al, 1993). There is an absence of flow related signal void.

Twenty-seven percent of these tumors extend into the middle and posterior cranial fossae. They usually

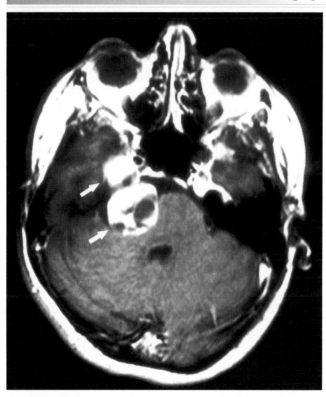

Figure 12.25

Axial T1W Gadolinium DTPA enhanced MRI scan showing a large right cystic trigeminal neuroma present in the middle and posterior cranial fossae (white arrows)

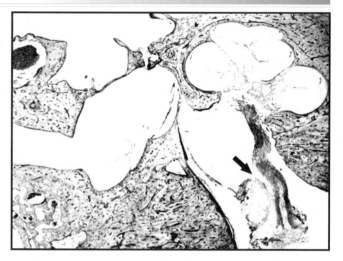

Figure 12.26

Histopathology of an arachnoid cyst in the IAC formed by splitting and duplication of the arachnoid layer (black arrow)

require a combined posterior and middle cranial fossa surgical approach. Anterior tumors require a Fisch type C inratemporal approach. Total resection may be difficult.

*Arachnoid cyst* Arachnoid cysts account for 0.7% of CPA tumors (Moffat et al, 1993) They are most commonly situated in the middle cranial fossa. They may occur in the CPA and/or IAC or over the convexity of the cerebellum.

Pathologically they are formed by splitting and duplication of the arachnoid layer. They are lined by arachnoid or ependyma and filled with cerebrospinal or xanthochromic fluid (Fig. 12.26). The large pseudo tumor variety may fill the CPA and erode bone. They may be congenital or aquired.

Congenital arachnoid cysts may remain clinically silent.

Acquired cysts arise from trauma or inflammation. They may be associated with intracranial extra-axial tumors.

Imaging reveals an enlarged IAC in more than 50% of cases.

CT scanning may be normal for small cysts. The lesion is hypodense with smooth edges. It does not enhance with intravenous contrast.

MRI reveals an hypointense lesion on T1 W images (Fig. 12.27) and markedly hyperintense image on T2W (Moffat et al, 1993).

Small cysts may never require treatment. In those requiring surgery complete excision of the cyst is not necessary. Decompression via a retrosigmoid approach is recommended. Smaller cysts may be decompressed via the retrolabyrinthine approach. Small cysts within the IAC can be tackled by a middle fossa approach.

*Metastases* Like arachnoid cysts they also comprise 0.7% of CPA lesions (Moffat et al, 1993). The symptoms and signs depend upon the site (Fig. 12.28). Primary tumors are most commonly of the breast and lung and also of the gastrointestinal and urinary tracts, or thyroid and sinuses.

Treatment is by palliative radiotherapy but local excision of solitary lesions can be remarkably beneficial.

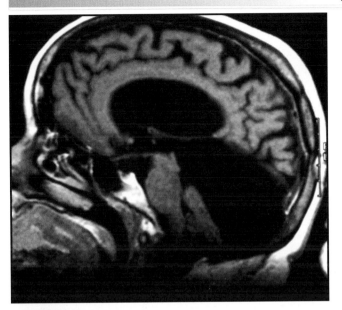

**Figure 12.27**

Sagittal T1W MRI scan of an arachnoid cyst. The lesion shows marked hypointensity

*Other cranial nerve neuromas*  The incidence of these neuromas is 0.2% (Moffat et al, 1993). The clinical features depend upon the nerve of origin. Histopathologically they are schwannomas and identical to acoustic neuromas.

CT and MRI features are the same as vestibular schwannoma but anatomical localization depends upon the nerve of origin. Glossopharyngeal and vagal neuromas are more inferior in the CPA and eccentric to the IAC (Fig. 12.29).

Surgery may require a combined transtemporal and retrosigmoid approach with resection of tumor in the skull base and neck.

*Lipoma*  Lipomas comprise 0.14% of CPA tumors (Moffat et al, 1993). Histopathologically they comprise mature fat cells (Fig. 12.30) and arise from embryological rests in the meninges. They differ from other intracranial lipomas in that they infiltrate cranial nerves

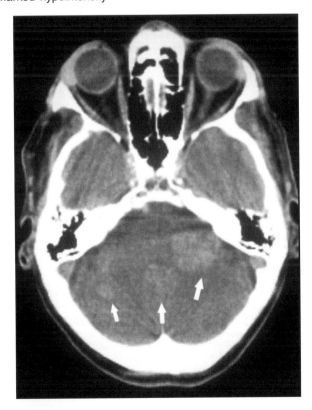

**Figure 12.28**

Axial CT revealing three hyperintense metastases secondary to prostatic carcinoma in the posterior cranial fossa (white arrows)

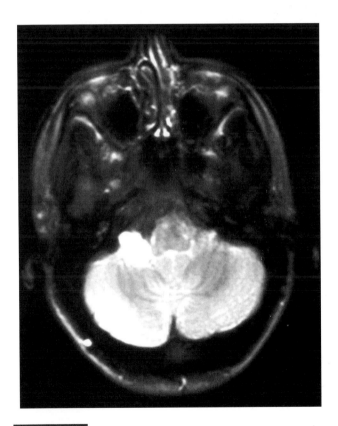

**Figure 12.29**

Axial Gadolinium DTPA enhanced T1W MRI of a glosso-pharyngeal neuroma eccentric from the IAC and inferior to it

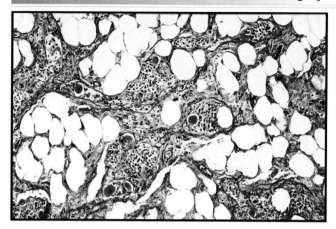

**Figure 12.30**

The histopathological features of a lipoma with mature fat cells clearly seen

and present with focal symptoms. The presenting symptoms and signs are similar to vestibular schwannomas (Monem et al, 1999). Facial weakness is not usually present.

CT scanning shows an homogeneous and very hypodense lesion which does not enhance.

The characteristic feature of a lipoma on MRI is a lesion of very high intensity on the *unenhanced* T1W image (Fig. 12.31) (Monem et al, *1999)*. There is no difference between the pre- and postcontrast images (Fig. 12.32). The lesion is also hyperintense on the T2W image. Fat suppressed images will markedly reduce the intensity of the lesion making the diagnosis.

These are usually indolent lesions many of which are not growing. They rarely require surgical resection and attempted surgery runs a high risk of facial nerve palsy.

*Cavernous hemangioma (extrinsic to facial nerve)* There are only a few reported cases in the CPA and IAC. Capillary hemangioma occurs in the temporal bone and may be an intrinsic facial nerve lesion. Cavernous hemangiomas may occur in the CPA (Fig. 12.33) or the IAC (Shaida et al, 2000)and mimic vestibular schwannoma.

Enlargement of the IAC is common.

CT scanning shows calcium stippling at high resolution. Intravenous contrast does not enhance the lesion.

MRI scanning reveals increased signal intensity on T1W (Fig. 12.34) and T2 W images (Moffat et al, 1993).

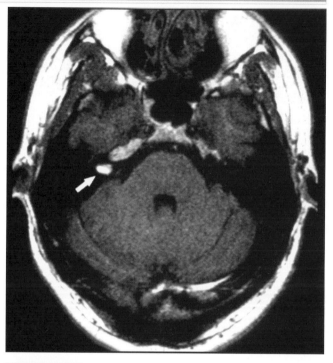

**Figure 12.31**

Axial unenhanced T1W MRI scan of a lipoma of the right IAC showing the markedly hyperintense lesion (white arrow)

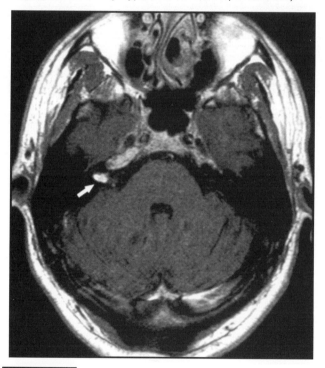

**Figure 12.32**

Axial contrast T1W scan of the same patient revealing that there is no difference between this and the unenhanced image (white arrow)

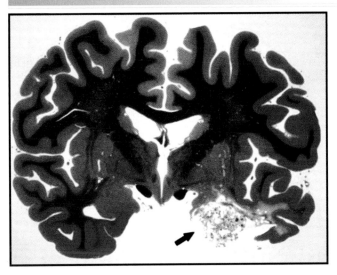

**Figure 12.33**

Coronal section through the brain showing the macroscopic features of a cavernous hemangioma

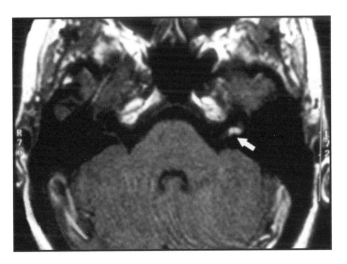

**Figure 12.34**

Axial T1W MRI scan of a small intracanalicular left sided hemangioma. Note the hyperintensity of the lesion on the unenhanced scan (white arrow)

*Arteriovenous (AV) malformation* These congenital lesions may be truly arteriovenous malformations or may arise due to a developmental venous anomaly (Moffat et al, 1993). They may occur in the CPA or on the dura where an audible bruit may be present. They rarely require treatment.

Dural AV malformations can be successfully treated by stereotactic radiotherapy and comprise a substantial proportion of all gamma knife treatments.

AV malformations in the CPA may spontaneously thrombose and largely disappear. They may be responsible for the enigmatic "disappearing CPA tumor" !! (Figs 12.35 to 12.37).

## Neurofibromatosis Type 2 (NF 2)

This is an autosomal dominant hereditary condition which may be devastating for the patient in its aggressive early onset Wishart type and still incapacitating in its less aggressive later in onset Gardiner type (Irving et al, 1997). It has the highest penetrance (95%) for an autosomal dominant. It usually arises from a gene deletion on the long arm of chromosome 22 at the locus of the amino acid sequence producing the protein merlin which is a tumor suppressor (Irving et al, 1994). Spontaneous mutations may be responsible for cases of NF2 without

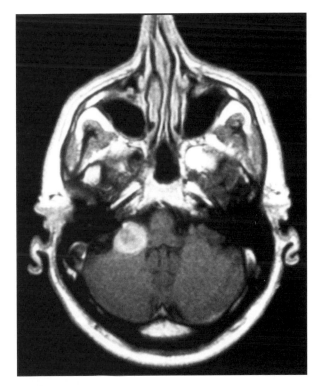

**Figure 12.35**

Axial T1W MRI scan of hyperintense thrombosed A-V malformation

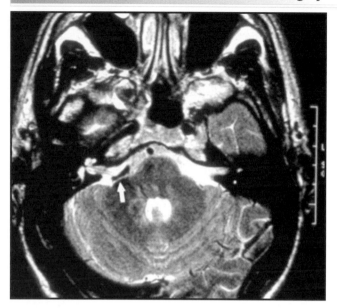

**Figure 12.36**
Axial T2W image of same lesion having almost disappeared 6 months later (white arrow)

a family history and sporadic mosaics may produce multiple but unilateral tumors. It is characterized by bilateral vestibular schwannomas with central and peripheral nerve tumors (Moffat et al, 1993). The patients often have multiple handicaps which may be bilateral. Its management poses one of the greatest challenges in modern skull base surgery.

The characteristic features of bilateral vestibular schwannomas (Fig. 12.38) are not infrequently associated with multiple meningiomas (Figs 12.39 and 12.40), low grade astrocytomas, ependymomas, gliomas, dermal fibromas, intrinsic (Fig. 12.40), and extrinsic spinal tumors other cranial nerve schwannomas and meningiomas as well as posterior subcapsular cataracts.

Rarely spectacular abdominal schwannomas are seen (Fig. 12.41).

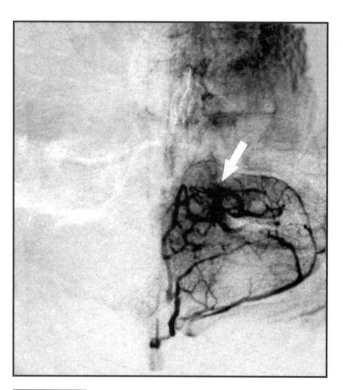

**Figure 12.37**
Venous phase of an arteriogram showing a developmental venous anomaly of the posterior cranial fossa (white arrow)

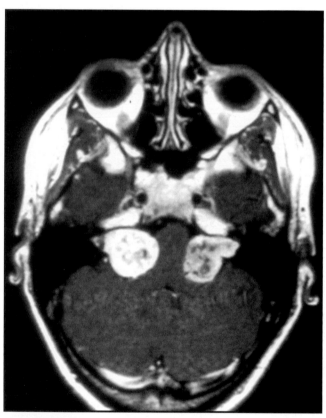

**Figure 12.38**
Gadolinium DTPA enhanced axial MRI scan showing bilateral large vestibular schwannomas in a patient with neurofibromatosis type 2(NF2)

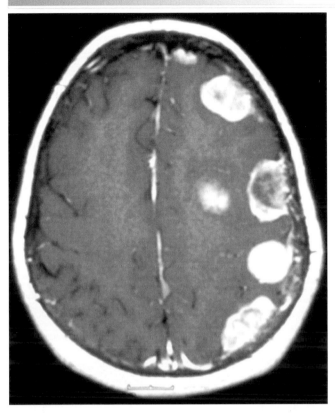

**Figure 12. 39**

Axial enhanced MRI scan demonstrating multiple meningiomas in a case of NF2

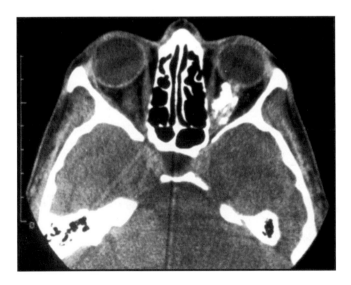

**Figure 12.40**

Axial CT of optic meningioma in the left orbit in a case of NF2

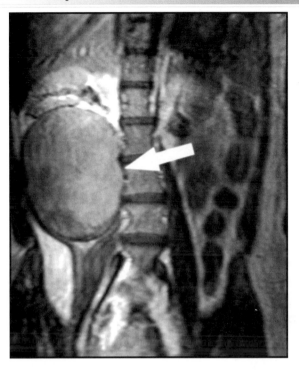

**Figure 12.41**

MRI scan of large abdominal neurofibroma in a case of NF2 (white arrow)

Intrinsic spinal lesions may be unresectable (Fig. 12.42).

The dilemmas in the management of this condition is polarized by the case illustrated in Figure 12.43 (Chang and Moffat, 2000). This 30-year old female presented with a small meningioma en plaque on the right side where she had no hearing and a total seventh nerve palsy. On the left side can be seen a very large cystic vestibular schwannoma with normal hearing. She had bilateral optic neuromas and was blind in the right eye. Thus, she only had hearing and eyesight on the side of this enormous lesion (Fig. 12.43).

The Cambridge surveillance protocol for NF2 consists of an annual MRI head scan and review in a multidisciplinary tertiary referral clinic which includes skull base and neurosurgeons, geneticists and counsellors. An initial MRI scan of the whole spine is followed by biannual scans in those patients with spinal tumors and repeat spinal scanning in those without only if suspicious neurological symptoms and signs emerge. Annual audiometry, both pure tone and

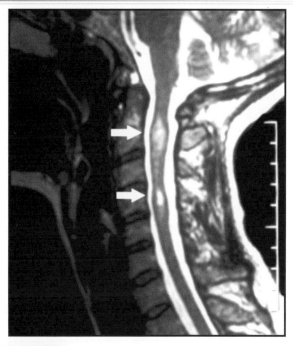

**Figure 12.42**

Sagittal T2W MRI scan of spinal cord showing intrinsic spinal lesions in NF2 (white arrows)

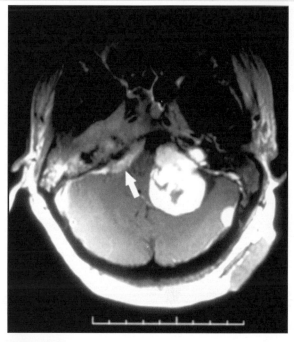

**Figure 12.43**

Axial T2W MRI scan of female patient aged 30 years with the Wishart type of NF2. Note the meningioma en plaque on the right (white arrow) where she had no hearing, a total facial palsy and a blind right eye due to bilateral optic gliomas. On the left side there is a large vestibular schwannoma where serviceable hearing is present

speech audiograms and regular ophthalmic examinations *are necessary.* (Evans et al, 2004– *In press*).

Management options (Moffat et al, 2002) include:

- Regular surveillance with interval imaging.
- Surgery to lesions causing threatening neurological compromise.
- Auditory brainstem implantation as a "***sleeper***" if inserted at the time of excision of the first vestibular schwannoma and certainly for the second side.
- Stereotactic radiotherapy has a limited place in the management of NF2. The results are not as good as in unilateral vestibular schwannoma and there is an increased risk of radiotherapy inducing malignant change in the tumor. Surgical excision of a tumor following stereotactic radiotherapy is associated with poor facial nerve results.

## LESIONS OF THE TEMPORAL BONE

### Cholesteatoma

Cholesteatoma of the temporal bone may be congenital or acquired.

### *Congenital Cholesteatoma*

Congenital cholesteatomas arise from embryonic undifferentiated cells which differentiate into squamous cells. Historically the term congenital cholesteatoma was reserved for those lesions of the cerebello-pontine angle and petrous apex (Fig. 12.44). Although there is argument about the possible role of such embryonic epidermoid cysts in the genesis of middle ear cholesteatoma most modern otologists and many pathologists believe this to be the case.

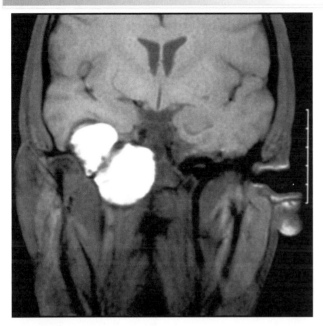

**Figure 12.44**

Coronal MRI scan showing a large CPA cholesteatoma

Cholesteatomas erode bone by three mechanisms:-
• Pressure on surrounding structures
• The secretion of osteolytic enzymes
• Osteitis due to surrounding granulation tissue

The latter is likely only to be associated with acquired cholesteatomas.

### Acquired Cholesteatoma

*Primary acquired cholesteatoma* refers to a lesion arising in the attic or postero-superior part of the middle ear, when there has been no previous history of otitis media. Initially, whatever their mode of origin, these may be uninfected, certainly so long as the keratin desquamated within them can be shed to the external ear canal. The disease may be silent at this stage but eventually the keratin becomes moist and infected. The effect of surface infection on the skin from which it has been shed is to encourage more desquamation and to impair surface migration, so that yet more infected keratin accumulates. This will actively erode bone.

*Secondary acquired cholesteatoma* follows active middle ear infection, usually with large postero-marginal defects of the tympanic membrane. Since this type of cholesteatoma is infected from the start it becomes apparent early because of foul smelling often scanty otorrhea.

These cholesteatomas erode bone and may therefore cause facial palsy.

CT scanning reveals a mass of soft tissue density and it is difficult to differentiate this from mucosal thickening or fibrosis. Smooth "*scalloped*" erosion of bone may make the otologist suspicious. Advances in imaging and higher resolution scanning as well as the utilization of MRI B1000 or diffusion weighted images is helpful in differential diagnosis and the concomitant management of the patient.

The propensity for extension of the cholesteatoma to invade the otic capsule and beyond to the petrous apex (Fig. 12. 45) (Atlas et al, 1992) makes imaging invaluable for surgical planning and patient counselling.

Involvement of the IAC may occur (Fig. 12.46) and this has great implications for the facial nerve, hearing and of course the risk of cerebro-spinal fluid leakage.

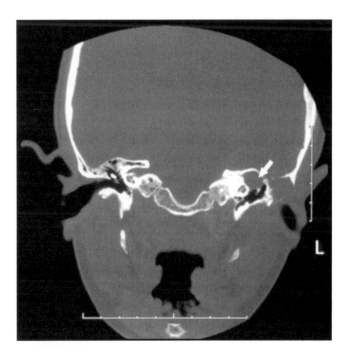

**Figure 12.45**

Coronal CT scan showing extensive cholesteatoma in the left temporal bone. It is involving the otic capsule (white arrow)

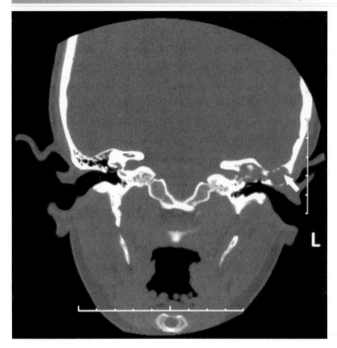

**Figure 12.46**

Coronal CT of same patient revealing cholesteatomatous erosion into the IAC

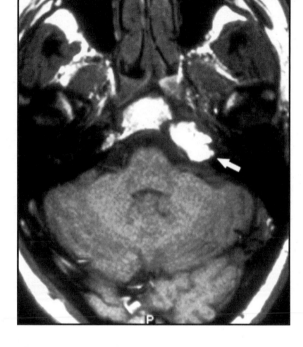

**Figure 12.47**

Axial T1W MRI scan showing an hyperintense cholesterol cyst of the petrous apex (white arrow)

## Cholesterol Granuloma

MRI helps in differentiating cholesteatoma from cholesterol granuloma (Moffat et al, 1993). In cholesteatoma the lesion is isointense or hypointense on the T1W image and hyperintense on the T2W image. In cholesterol granuloma the lesion is hyperintense on both the T1W and T2W images (Figs 12.47 and 12.48).

In this patient there is a bony defect in the middle fossa plate clearly seen on the coronal CT (Fig. 12.49).

The MRI scan shows what we have described as the "*billiard pocket sign*"(Quaranta et al, 2002). On the coronal T1W image there is an area of hypointensity at the level of the middle fossa defect and also just superior to it in the middle fossa and above this an area of hyperintensity. Presumably this represents cholesteatoma extending through the middle fossa defect with an associated cholesterol containing cyst (Figs 12.50 and 12.51).

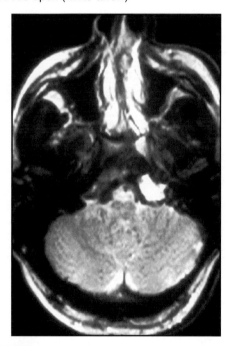

**Figure 12.48**

Axial T2W MRI scan demonstrating that the lesion is also hyperintense on the T2W image

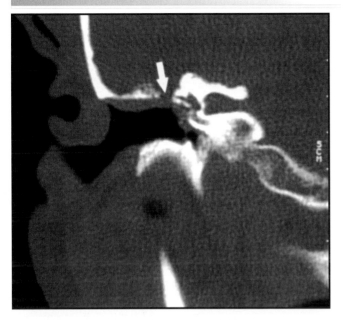

**Figure 12.49**

Coronal CT scan of a patient with a cholesteatoma eroding through the middle fossa plate on the right side (white arrow)

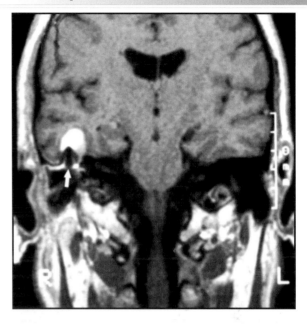

**Figure 12.51**

Coronal view in the same patient with an hypointense area in the region of the defect and an hyperintense area superior to this (white arrow)

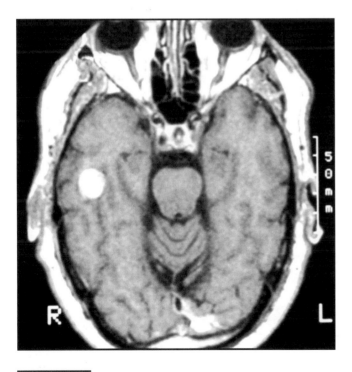

**Figure 12.50**

Axial T1W MRI scan with an hyperintense lesion in the right middle cranial fossa

## Malignant Otitis Externa

This rare condition which may occur in diabetics produces a slowly expanding inflammatory granulomatous erosion of the temporal bone which may extend and affect any of the structures in the temporal bone and CPA. A mass of soft tissue density with irregular erosion of bone are the features on CT. A lesion of high signal intensity is seen on MR imaging. Indium labelled white cell scans will delineate the "*hot spot*" in the temporal bone and possibly the CPA. Loss of hearing, facial palsy and palsies of the last few cranial nerves may occur.

## Wegener's Granulomatosis

The characteristic vasculitis in this condition tends to produce similar appearances on imaging to malignant otitis externa.

## Tumors of the Temporal Bone

Benign

## Glomus Jugulare Tumors

Fisch type A, B and C involve the temporal bone but not the CPA (see lesions of CPA). The characteristic symptoms and signs and the features on imaging have already been described. A pulsatile mass in the middle ear may be caused by:

• Glomus tumors
• Lateral aberrant carotid artery
• High jugular bulb
• Middle ear adenoma

These comprise the differential diagnosis (Moffat et al, 1989) and it is particularly important to exclude a lateral aberrant carotid artery (Fig. 12.52) and high jugular bulb (Fig. 12.53) in the management of these patients.

The "rising sun sign" may be seen in all of these conditions but typically in glomus tympanicum and glomus jugulare tumors (Fig. 12.54).

Glomus tympanicum tumors are confined to the middle ear (Fig. 12.54), arise out of the hypotympanum and do not erode the bone of the dome of the jugular bulb (Fig. 12.55) (Moffat et al, 1993).

Glomus jugulare tumors types, B, C and D erode the jugular foramen (Figs 12.56 and 12.57).

In non- chromaffin paragangliomas high resolution CT scanning delineates the exact extent of the bony erosion and MRI has the advantage of defining the soft tissue tumor mass in multiplanar images and allows

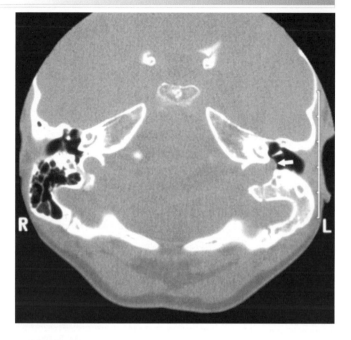

**Figure 12.53**

Axial CT of high jugular bulb on the left side (white arrow)

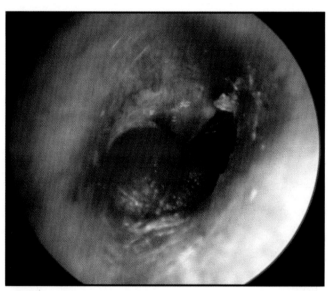

**Figure 12.54**

Otoscopic view of "rising sun sign" seen in a glomus jugulare tumor

assessment of the state of the carotid artery and defines intracranial extension (Fig. 12.58).

Extension into the neck (Figs 12.59 and 12.60) may erode the cervical vertebrae particularly in more

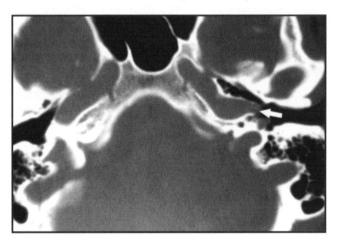

**Figure 12.52**

Axial CT of temporal bones demonstrating an aberrant carotid artery on the left side (white arrow)

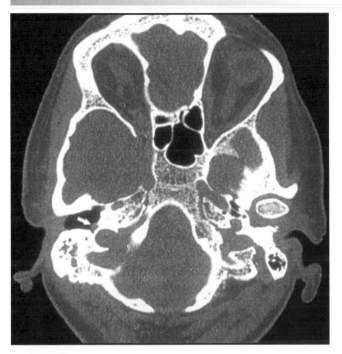

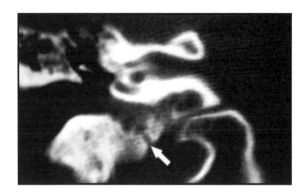

**Figure 12.57**

Coronal CT with middle ear opacification due to a mass of soft tissue density eroding the dome of the jugular bulb (white arrow). This is another example of a glomus jugulare tumor

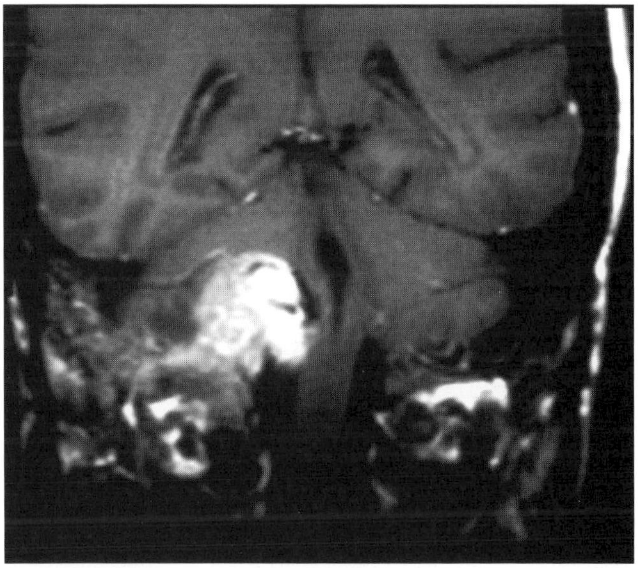

**Figure 12.55**

Axial CT scan of right glomus tympanicum tumor (Fisch type A). There is no erosion of the jugular bulb (white arrow)

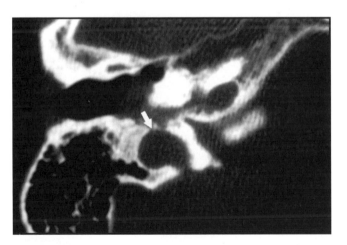

**Figure 12.56**

Axial CT of glomus jugulare tumor on right side with erosion of the bone of the jugular bulb (white arrow)

**Figure 12.58**

Coronal T1W MRI scan of enormous Fisch type Di2 glomus jugulare tumor with marked brainstem compression and shift of the fourth ventricle

aggressive tumors which tend to occur in the younger patient.

Carotid arteriography is still important for screening for concurrent, multicentric lesions, for defining the principle feeding vessels, the size and patency of the contralateral lateral sinus and purposes of pre-operative or pre-radiotherapeutic embolization.

Figure 12.61 is a carotid arteriogram of a carotid body tumor showing the "*lyre bird sign*" because the appearance is similar to the tail of a lyre bird.

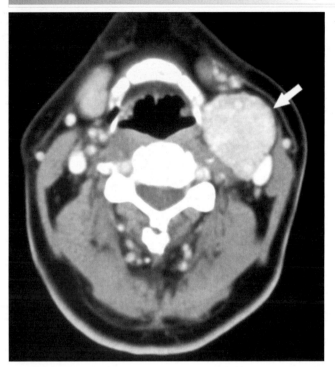

**Figure 12.59**

Axial CT scan of the neck revealing the presence of a large soft tissue mass which is a glomus tumor (white arrow)

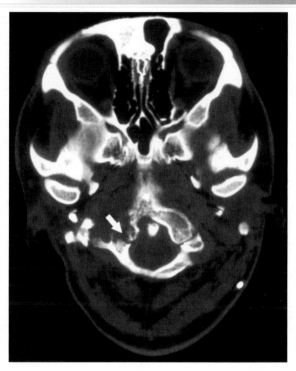

**Figure 12.60**

Axial CT scan of the neck showing erosion of a cervical vertebra by a large glomus tumor in a young patient (white arrow)

## Carcinoid

Carcinoid tumors (argentaffinoma) of the temporal bone are incredibly rare. The small round, darkly staining cells are arranged in solid clumps or cylinders and acinar differentiation is unusual. If the cells are fixed freshly in formalin, special granules can be demonstrated with silver stains. Some carcinoid tumors are secreting and are associated with an endocrine syndrome characterized by episodic flushing, diarrhea, breathlessness and occasionally organic pulmonary stenosis. They are associated with the secretion of serotonin. They are benign tumors that pursue a very indolent course. CT scanning here in the axial plane reveals opacification with a mass of soft tissue density (Fig. 12.62). There is no bone destruction.

Glomus jugulare and carcinoid tumors look identical on imaging but have different immuno-histochemical characteristics which differentiate them.

- Granular cell tumors
- Giant cell tumors

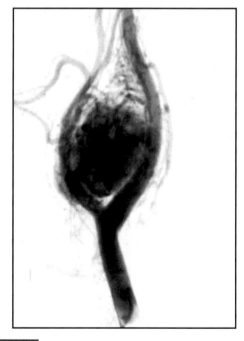

**Figure 12.61**

Carotid body tumor producing the "lyre bird sign" on carotid arteriography

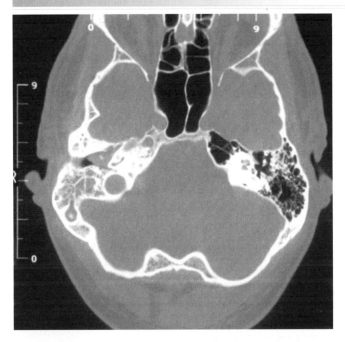

**Figure 12.62**

Axial CT scan of a patient with a carcinoid tumor of the temporal bone. This presents as a mass of soft tissue density with no erosion of the bony trabeculae

- Adenoma
- Extradural meningioma

All these tumors are benign and patients present with a mass of soft tissue density in the temporal bone. They are distinguished histopathologically.

## Tumors of the Temporal Bone

*Primary malignant*

## Squamous Carcinoma

These difficult very aggressive malignant tumors of the temporal bone have a very poor prognosis and a low 5-year survival (Moffat et al, 1997). They have an incidence of 0.8 per million per year in males and are slightly more common in females with an incidence of 1 per million.

An exophytic, bleeding, painful mass in the external auditory canal (Fig. 12.63) or middle ear/mastoid are the characteristic features and facial nerve palsy may be a relatively early sign.

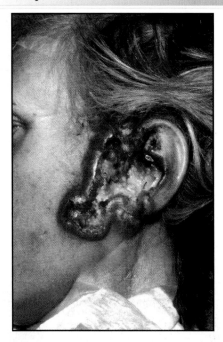

**Figure 12.63**

Appearance of an advanced squamous carcinoma (SCC) of the temporal bone. Note the ulcerated fungating tumor with rolled edges

They have a propensity to spread superiorly through the tegmen or middle fossa plate (Fig. 12.64) and may invade dura (Fig. 12.65) and subsequently the temporal lobe of the brain.

In order to improve the 5-year survival these tumors need radical excision by an extended temporal bone resection (Figs 12.66 to 12.68) with flap repair of the defect and postoperative radiotherapy (Moffat and Wagstaff 2003).

In the elderly a very long procedure should be avoided and a scalp rotation flap may be necessary. Free flap repair is very successful in the younger patient and the "modified Chinese flap" based on the anterior cubital artery (Figs 12.69 to 12.71) rather than the classical distal radial flap has been applied very successfully.

Free trapezius, antero-lateral fore-arm and antero-lateral thigh free flaps have been used more recently in the series and have the advantage that the donor site can be closed primarily and does not require split skin grafting (Moffat and Wagstaff 2002).

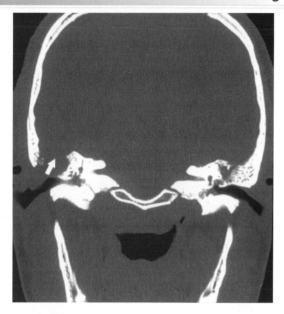

**Figure 12.64**

Coronal CT of SCC of temporal bone. There is marked erosion of the middle fossa plate and extension into the middle cranial fossa (white arrow)

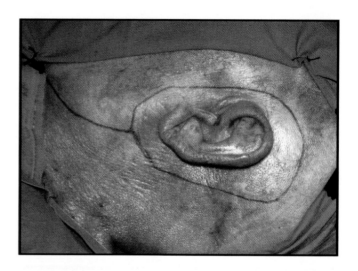

**Figure 12.66**

Incision for extended temporal bone resection for SCC of temporal bone. An oval 10 × 8 cm is marked out on the skin with a tail into the neck in a skin crease

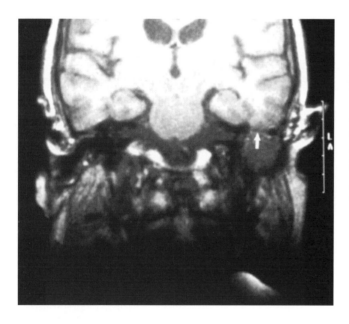

**Figure 12.65**

Coronal T1W MRI scan of SCC of left temporal bone eroding into the middle cranial fossa and involving the dura and temporal lobe (white arrow)

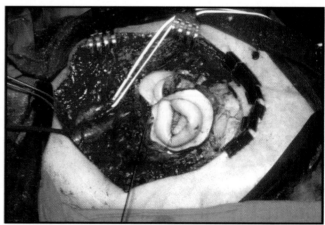

**Figure 12.67**

Slings are placed around the great vessels to obtain vascular control and the whole temporal bone is excised along with the head of the mandible, glenoid fossa, ascending ramus of mandible and a total parotidectomy is also performed. It may be necessary to excise involved dura widely and also a part of the temporal lobe of the brain if this is involved by tumor. The venous sinus and the ninth, tenth and eleventh cranial nerves may also have to be sacrificed to obtain a clear margin

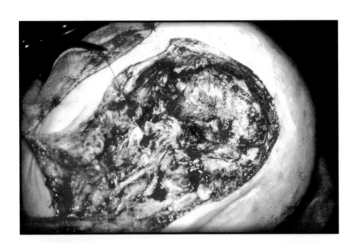

**Figure 12.68**

This is the surgical defect after the resection. The dural defects are grafted with fascia lata and the wedge shaped defect is obliterated with fat and fascia lata prior to flap repair

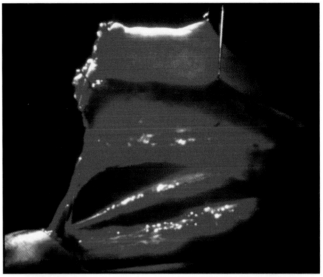

**Figure 12.70**

Transillumination of the vascular pedicle

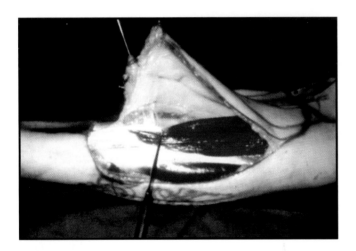

**Figure 12.69**

Modified Chinese flap based on the anterior cubital artery being raised

Prosthetic ears can produce remarkable cosmesis but in some climates require a summer and a winter ear (Figs 12.72 and 12.73).

## Tumors of the Temporal Bone

*Secondary malignant* Secondary tumors in the temporal bone are present in 27% of patients with

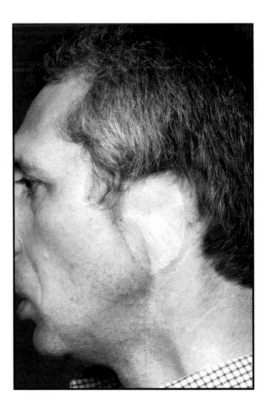

**Figure 12.71**

The excellent cosmetic result of the free flap repair

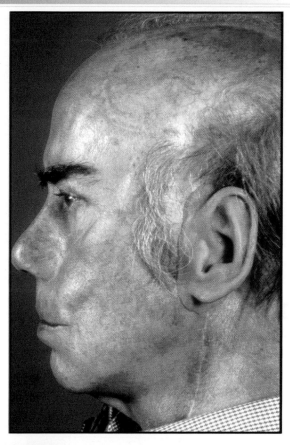

**Figure 12.72**

Prosthetic ear has to be glued in place since there is no bone to osseo-integrate a titanium post. This is the summer ear

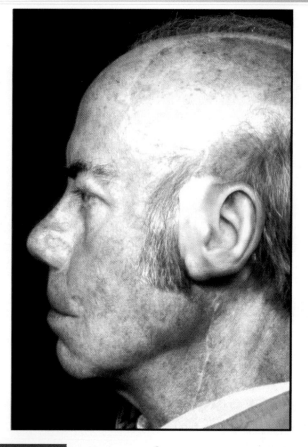

**Figure 12.73**

In many climates a winter ear is required since there is no bone to osseo-integrate a titanium post. This is the winter ear

advanced malignancy (Figs 12.74 and 12.75) (Moffat et al, 1993). They are usually overshadowed by the primary growth and other metastatic lesions. The endochondral layer of the bone is resistant to invasion. The most common sites of origin are:
- Breast
- Kidney
- Lung
- Stomach
- Larynx
- Prostate
- Thyroid

The most common sites for metastatic involvement of the temporal bone are:
- IAC
- Mastoid portion
- Tympanic portion
- Labyrinthine portion

## Lesions of the Parotid

These may affect the pes anserinus or the distal intraparotid portion of the facial nerve.

### Tumors of the Parotid

*Primary malignant* Eighty percent of occult primary lesions of the parotid are malignant (Fig. 12.76 ). Non-malignant lesions can produce a facial palsy due to pressure, kinking, inflammation and local toxic effects.

### Surgical Approaches for Facial Nerve Palsy

The surgical approach depends upon the pathology, its site and extent and the results of high resolution imaging. The following surgical approaches may be utilized:
- Translabyrinthine
- Transcochlear

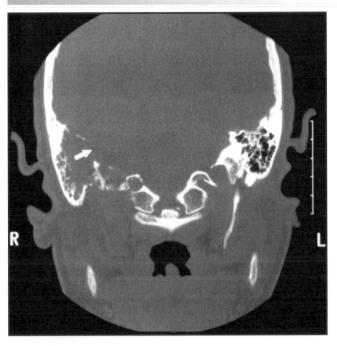

**Figure 12.74**

The soft tissue mass eroding the right temporal bone is due to a metastasis and can be seen on this axial CT scan (white arrow)

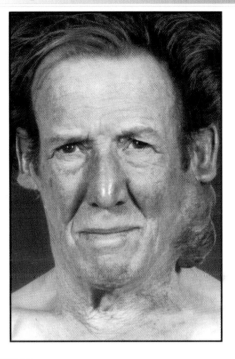

**Figure 12.76**

Large malignant adenoid cystic carcinoma of the parotid salivary gland

- Retrosigmoid
- Middle fossa
- Transmastoid
- Transmastoid-middle cranial fossa.
- Infratemporal
- Lateral/subtotal/total petrosectomy
- Parotidectomy

It is useful to adopt a combination of approaches in some instances.

### Facial Nerve Rehabilitation

If more than 75% of the nerve can be preserved intact then recovery is likely to be satisfactory and at least a House Brackmann Grade III (Fig. 12.77) can be achieved with good eye closure. If more than 25% of the nerve is damaged it may be better to consider excision of the damaged segment with primary anastomosis if enough length can be obtained by taking the nerve out of the fallopian canal. If not or if a large segment of the nerve has to be excised then it

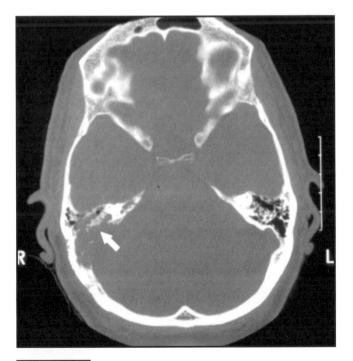

**Figure 12.75**

The coronal CT image clearly demonstrates the extent of the bone erosion(white arrow)

117

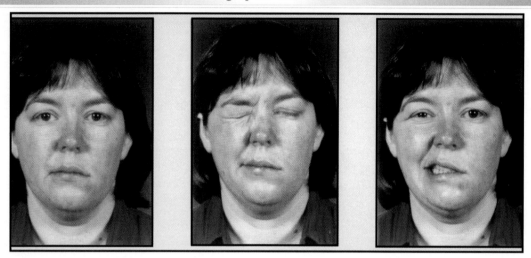

**Figure 12.77**

House-Brackmann grade III facial palsy

may be necessary to consider grafting with greater auricular or sural nerve.

## CONCLUSIONS

A total facial palsy is a very significant neurological deficit which leads to a considerable reduction in the patient's quality of life. This chapter has described in detail the presenting symptoms and signs and findings on imaging of all the interesting tumors which may *result in a facial palsy* throughout the length of the facial nerve. The surgical approaches which may be considered to excise the various pathologies have been mentioned but not described in detail since this was not the remit of this chapter. The clinical aspects of these tumors have been presented and are based on the author's own experience in the Department of Otoneurological and Skull Base Surgery at Cambridge University Hospital over the last 23 years.

## BIBLIOGRAPHY

1. Altlas MD, Moffat DA, Hardy DG: Petrous apex cholesteatoma: Diagnostic and treatment dilemmas. Laryngoscope 1992;102:1363-68.
2. Baguley DM, Moffat D, Tsui YN: Audiological findings in medial and lateral acoustic neuromas. British Journal of Audiology 1989;23;2:158-59.
3. Baguley DM, Beynon GJ, Grey PL, Hardy DG, Moffat DA: Audio-vestibular findings in CPA Meningioma. Proceedings of the 2nd International Conference on Acoustic Neuroma and 2nd European Skull Base Society Congress, Paris, April 22-26, 1995. Edited by JM Sterkers, R Charachon and O Sterklers Kugler Publications, Amsterdam/New York/Paris 1995;95-97.
4. Beynon GJ, Baguley DM, Moffat DA, Irving RM: Positional vertigo as a first symptom of a cerebellopontine angle cholesteatoma: A case report. Ear Nose and Throat Journal 2000;79(7):508-11.
5. Brewis C, Bottrill ID, Wharton SB, Moffat DA: Glomus jugulare tumor with metastases to cervical lymph nodes. Journal of Laryngology and Otology 2000;114(1):67-69.
6. Chang P, Moffat DA: Neurofibromatosis Type 2: A 15-year experience and current review. Australian Journal of Otolaryngology 2000;3(5):528-42.
7. Evans DGR, Baser M O'Reilly, B Rowe, J Gleeson, M Saeed, S King et al: Management of the patient and family with neurofibromatosis type 2: A consensus conference statement. Lancet, in press, 2003.
8. Grey PL, Moffat DA, Hardy DG, Baguley DM, Beynon GJ. Audio-vestibular results after surgery for cerebello-pontine meningiomas. American Journal of Otology 1996;17(4): 634-38.
9. Harada T, Irving RM, Moffat DA, Hardy DG, Xuereb JH, Barton DE, et al: Molecular Genetic Investigation of meningioma. Human Molecular Genetics 1995;3(2):347-50.
10. Hardy DG, Macfarlane R, Baguley DM, Moffat DA: Surgery for acoustic neuroma: An analysis of one hundred translabyrinthine operations. Journal of Neurosurgery 1989;71:799-804.

11. Hardy DG, Macfarlane R, Baguley DM, Moffat DA: Facial nerve recovery following acoustic neuroma surgery. British Journal of Neurosurgery 1989;3:675-80.

12. Irving RM, Moffat DA, Hardy DG, Barton DE, Xuereb JH, Maher ER: Somatic NF2 gene mutations in familial and non-familial vestibular schwannoma. Human Molecular Genetics 1994;3(2):347-50.

13. Irving RM, Harada T, Moffat DA, Hardy DG, Whittaker JL, Maher ER: Somatic neurofibromatosis Type 2 gene mutations and growth characteristics in vestibular schwannoma. American Journal of Otology 1997;18(6):754-60.

14. Moffat DA, Saunders JE, McElveen JT, McFerran D, Hardy DG: Unusual cerebello-pontine angle tumors. Journal of Laryngology and Otology 1993;107:1087-98.

15. Moffat DA, Croxson GR, Baguley DM, Hardy DG: Brun's Bidirectional Nystagmus in Cerebellopontine Tumors. Clinical Otolaryngology 1988;13(1):153-15.

16. Moffat DA, Hardy DG, Baguley DM: The strategy and benefits of acoustic neuroma searching. Journal of Laryngology and Otology 1989;103:51-59.

17. Moffat DA, Hardy DG: Surgical management of large glomus jugulare tumors: The infra and transtemporal approach. Journal of Laryngology and Otology 1989;103:1167-80.

18. Moffat DA, Irving RM, Hardy DG: Sudden deafness in acoustic neuroma. Journal of Laryngology and Otology 1994;108(2):116-19.

19. Moffat DA, Ballagh RH: Rare tumors of the cerebellopontine angle. Clinical Oncology of The Royal College of Radiologists 1995;7(1):28-41.

20. Moffat DA, Hardy DG, Grey PL, Baguley DM: The operative learning curve and its effect on facial nerve outcome in vestibular schwannoma surgery. American Journal of Otology 1996;17(4):643-47.

21. Moffat DA, Baguley DM, Beynon GJ, da Cruz M: Clinical acumen and vestibular schwannoma. American Journal of Otology 1998;19:288-91.

22. Moffat DA: Moffat Classification of Facial Nerve Function. A Supplemental Issue for The 11th Keio University international Symposium for Life Sciences and Medicine. Consensus Meeting on Systems for Reporting Results in Acoustic Neuroma. Keio Journal of Medicine 2001;50(Suppl 4):38-39.

23. Moffat DA, Quaranta N, Baguley DM, Hardy DG, Chang P: Management strategies in neurofibromatosis type 2. European Archives of Otorhinolaryngology 2002;260:12-18.

24. Moffat DA, Quaranta N, Baguley DM, Hardy DG, Moffat DA: Staging and management of primary cerebellopontine cholesteatoma. Journal of Laryngology and Otology 2002;116:340-45.

25. Moffat DA, Wagstaff SA: Squamous cell carcinoma of the temporal bone. Current Opinion in Otolaryngology and Head and Neck Surgery 2003;11(2):107-11.

26. Monem SA, Chiossone-Kerdel JA, Moffat DA: Lipoma of the cerebellopontine angle; a case report. In Sanna M, Taibah A, Russo A, Mancini F (Eds): Proceedings of the Third International conferenrce on Acoustic Neuroma and other CXPA Tumors Monduzzi Editore, S.p.A. Bologna 1999;823-30.

27. Quaranta N, Chang P, Moffat DA: Unusual MRI appearance of an intracranial cholesteatoma extension; The "billiard pocket sign". Ear Nose and Throat Journal 2002;81(9):645-47.

28. Quaranta N, Baguley DM, Axon PR, Moffat DA: Conservative Management of Vestibular Schwannomas. In Baguley DM, Ramsden RT, Moffat DA (Eds): Fourth International Conference on Vestibular Schwannoma and other CPA Lesions. Conference Proceedings. Immediate Proceedings Ltd 2003;256-57.

29. Quaranta N, Chang P, Baguley DM, Moffat DA. Audiological Presentation of Cerebellopontine Angle Cholesteatoma. Journal of Otolaryngology 2003;32(4):217-21.

30. Shaida AM, McFerran DJ, da Cruz M, Moffat DA, Hardy DG: Cavernous haemangioma of the internal auditory canal. Journal of Laryngology and Otology 2000;114(6):453-55.

❉ ❉ ❉ ❉

# CHAPTER 13
# Plastic-surgical Repair of the Paralyzed Face

*Narendra Pandya, Ashok Shah*

## INTRODUCTION

The face plays a very important role in communication. In facial nerve paralysis, the face is paralyzed and all expressions are lost. The patient loses the power of communication, develops an inferiority complex and is depressed. Facial paralysis results in severe psychological, cosmetic and functional disabilities.

The goals in the treatment of facial paralysis are to achieve normal appearance at rest, symmetry with voluntary motion as well as with involuntary emotional control of the ocular, oral, and nasal sphincters and no significant functional deficit secondary to the reconstructive surgery (Grabb and Smith, 1997). Functional recovery takes priority in the reconstruction. It is of utmost importance, in view of the possibility of corneal ulceration and blindness, to prevent eye complications in the patient with facial paralysis. The treatment of facial paralysis requires the skill of many specialties like neurosurgeon, neurologist, ophthalmologist, otolaryngologist, and plastic surgeon. A multiple or combined surgical approach depending on the cause, time interval, and wound characteristics often gives best results.

A wide range of procedures is available but the totally paralyzed face can never be made normal by any of the modern and recent surgical methods of reconstruction. The surgeon must employ a number of concepts depending on the etiology, the time interval, the wound characteristics, and the availability and necessity of neuromuscular substitution. No single surgical method can correct a complex deformity, and results of surgery are not always gratifying (Mahaluxmivala, 1998).

## ANATOMY

A fundamental knowledge of the surgical anatomy of the parotid gland and facial nerve is essential for the surgeon reconstructing patients with facial paralysis. In infants, the facial nerve lies more superficially.

### Intratemporal Facial Nerve

The facial nerve is formed by supranuclear and infranuclear fibres from the facial nucleus. It leaves the pons and enters the facial canal of the temporal bone. The facial nerve gives greater superficial petrosal nerve, (supplies secretomotor fibres to the lacrimal gland, taste sensations from the soft palate), nerve to the stapedius muscle (sound vibrations) and chorda tympani nerve (provides secretomotor fibres to the submaxillary and sublingual glands, and taste fibres from the anterior two-third of the tongue).

### Extratemporal Facial Nerve

The larger superficial segment of the parotid gland lies lateral to the facial nerve branches, and the smaller deep portion lies medial to these branches. The facial nerve emerges from the skull through the stylomastoid foramen, gives muscular rami to various muscles and enters the parotid gland. In the parotid gland, the nerve splits into two main divisions, the temporofacial and the cervicofacial portions. The two divisions sub-branch to form five main branches: the temporal, zygomatic, buccal, mandibular, and cervical. These branches supply the muscles of facial expression.

## ETIOLOGY AND CLASSIFICATION

The various etiologic factors involved may be broadly classified into three major groups: intracranial, intra-temporal, and extracranial.

### Intracranial

- Vascular abnormalities
- CNS degenerative diseases
- Intracranial tumors
- Trauma to the brain
- Congenital abnormalities and agenesis

### Intratemporal

- Bacterial and viral infections
- Trauma
- Tumors invading the middle ear, mastoid, and facial nerve

### Extracranial

- Parotid tumors
- Trauma
- Malignant tumors of the mandible, pterygoid region, and skin

## EVALUATION

A careful history is obtained, including the onset and duration of the condition and the degree of recovery. Various topognostic tests like hearing test, balance tests, Schimer test, stapes reflex, submandibular flow test, and taste tests are done. Additionally, the physician examines the face at rest and in motion, noting muscular tone and symmetry and analyzing the various mimetic muscles. Motor function is tested by asking the patient to wrinkle the forehead, close the eyelids tightly, show the teeth, pucker the lips, and grimace. The platysma muscle and depressors can be tested by having the patient draw the lower lip and angle of the mouth downward. Paralysis of the buccinator and orbicularis oris muscles results in speech impairment, drooling, and inability to whistle or puff out the cheeks.

Various electro-diagnostic tests of facial nerve and muscles are performed to establish a physiologic baseline of neuromuscular status (Mahaluxmivala, 1998). Tomographic, angiographic, and neurological investigations add valuable information about intratemporal lesions.

## LOCATION OF THE LESION

Supranuclear paralysis involves only paralysis of the lower facial muscles contralateral to the side of the lesion. Lesions in the pons, intratemporal, or extra-temporal portion, result in weakness of the entire ipsilateral half of the face, including the forehead. Intra-temporal lesions can be identified by Schimer's test (lacrimal gland function), intolerance to loud sound (stapedius branch), and applying galvanic current and noting metallic taste on normal side and electric shock on affected side of the tongue. In extratemporal lesion, patient loses movements of facial muscles and facial expressions.

## CHOICE OF PROCEDURE

Dynamic reconstruction and neural reconstruction are almost always preferred to static methods, except under special circumstances (McCarthy, 1990). Two essential elements are required for facial movement: an intact facial nerve and functional facial muscles. If the facial muscles are healthy, the requirements for reinnervation are:

1. A viable ipsilateral facial nerve nucleus
2. A proximal nerve segment capable of supporting axonal regeneration, and
3. A distal nerve segment through which axons may regenerate to the facial muscles.

However, significant muscular degeneration may preclude reanimation without the transfer of new muscular tissue to the face. Lacerations and iatrogenic injuries of the facial nerve are best repaired immediately. It is within the first three weeks after injury that the neural and muscular elements have the best chance of complete recovery. Muscles degenerate after 1 to 2 years of paralysis but they are capable of functioning again if the regenerating nerve reaches them, i.e. via nerve grafting or nerve crossover procedure, which are the procedures of choice. If the muscle is not rein-nervated, it undergoes atrophy with disappearance of contractile elements. There is often a combination of neural and muscular deficit requiring transfer of both elements for reanimation. After two years muscles degenerate hence muscle transfer or static reconstruction are more suitable techniques (McCarthy, 1990).

## TREATMENT

### Aims

1. Full function of the face at rest and during expression, but this is rarely achieved.
2. Symmetry of oral fissure.
3. Control of oral and ocular sphincter function, and
4. Spontaneous and natural expression of emotions.

Reconstruction can be either dynamic or static.

### *Dynamic Reconstruction*

*Neural repair:*

1. *Direct nerve repair and grafting:* The most effective means of rehabilitating the paralyzed face is to reestablish the neural pathway by direct approximation or autogenous nerve grafting. Each of these approaches requires adequate mimetic muscle function. Usually good results are obtained up to one year following facial paralysis. Direct nerve approximation is indicated in any instance in which the main trunk can be reapproximated with no tension (Grabb and Smith, 1997). However, immediate facial nerve grafting is used to overcome loss of the main trunk, peripheral branches, or a nerve segment. Obviously, if the distal part of the facial nerve including the mimetic muscles is ablated, nerve grafting is unrealistic; muscle transposition is the preferred treatment in such cases.

Branches from the cervical plexus from the ipsilateral or contralateral side are most frequently used for facial nerve autografting and they are sutured to the terminal branches of the temporal, zygomatic, buccal, and mandibular divisions. The sural nerve is an alternative donor site. The nerve graft should be sutured without any tension and it should lie in a healthy, well-vascularized area

free of scar tissue. The fascicular repair with atraumatic technique by using operating microscope gives the best results and the timing of repair is of utmost importance, the ideal situation being at the time of the primary ablative procedure. The time interval for return of facial movement varies from 6-24 months, depending on the length of the graft. The quality of return is always mass movement. There is always a deficit in emotional expression.

2. *Cross-face nerve grafting (Facio-facial anastomoses):* The procedure is based on cross-innervations from the non-paralyzed side by means of sural nerve grafts that connect the reservoir of peripheral healthy facial nerve fascicles to the corresponding branches of specific muscle groups on the paralyzed side (Cohen, 1994).

Fascicular repair is used and the length of the grafts varies from 6 to 8 cm. Most authors prefer a two-stage procedure, allowing the nerve axons to grow to the opposite side, and then resecting the neuroma to demonstrate the success of the axon regrowth before suturing the graft to the paralyzed side. This procedure has limited applications (except when combined with micro-neuromuscular muscle transfers) and the overall results were disappointing when compared to those obtained with classic procedures.

*Operative technique:* In this the buccal branches of the facial nerve on the nonparalyzed side is sutured microsurgically to the corresponding branches of the facial nerve on the paralyzed side (or to the nerve of a vascularized muscle) by using the sural nerve graft. This procedure is done in two stages.

Sacrifice of facial nerve branches, on the normal side does not produce long-term weakness and may even be beneficial in equalizing the two sides.

The primary disadvantage is long operating time and the time required for return of function. The facial muscles undergo further atrophy during the time required for axonal growth through the long nerve grafts. The greatest disadvantage of this technique is that only 50% of all nerve fibres of the facial nerve can be used from the normal side, and they are joined to about 50% of the paralyzed side, thereby limiting the amount of axonal input.

In general, the distinct disadvantages include the following:

1. There are two suture lines for each nerve graft, increasing the probability of a greater loss of sprouting axons.
2. A longer time is required for reinnervation from these long grafts, during which there may be further muscle atrophy.
3. The greatest disadvantage is the reduced axonal input to accomplish powerful rein-nervation if one is not to sacrifice too much function on the normal side.
4. Technical difficulty in identifying distal branches of the facial nerve.
5. Postoperatively mass movements are seen.

The cross-face nerve graft is only another alternative to the classic procedures of hypoglossal facial nerve crossover and muscle transposition.

3. *Nerve crossover:* The surgical technique is straightforward and has the advantage of requiring only one anastomosis of nerves that are a satisfactory physical match. (McCarthy , 1990).

Nerve crossovers are used when direct anasto-moses or grafting is not feasible when facial paralysis is resulting from intracranial lesions or disorders of the temporal bone. Commonly used nerves are glossopharyngeal, accessory, phrenic, and hypoglossal nerves. The hypoglossal-facial nerve crossover is the most popular crossover operation in use today.

Nerve crossover techniques are advantageous because they are simple, require only a single suture line, and serve as a powerful source of innervations. The main disadvantage is that they result in associated, uncoordinated movements, loss of emotion on face, and in loss of function of the donor nerve.

*Muscle repair:*

1. *Muscle transfers:* Transfer of muscle to the paralyzed face is usually done under following circumstances.
   a. After long-standing muscle atrophy.
   b. As an adjunct to the mimetic muscles to pro-vide new muscle and myoneurotization, and
   c. In combination with a nerve graft or crossover nerve implanted in the transposed muscle. Masseter and temporalis muscle transposition are most commonly used.

*Masseter muscle transposition* (Fig. 13.1): This muscle is ideally suited to give motion to the lower half of the face (De Castro and Zani, 1993). Commonly, three muscle slips are sutured to the dermis of the lower lip, oral commissure, and upper lip. Over-correction must be accomplished. The patient maintains voluntary control over the muscle and can activate it by clenching the teeth.

*Temporalis muscle transposition* (Figure 13.2): For facial rehabilitation, the temporalis muscle has

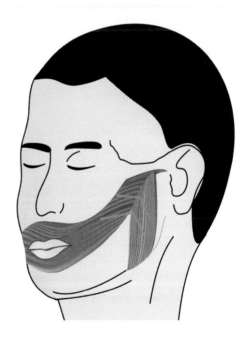

**Figure 13.1**

Masseter muscle transposition

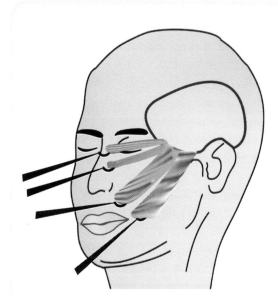

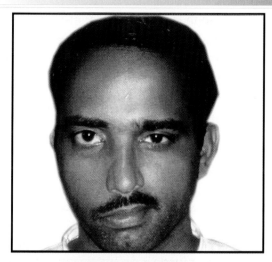

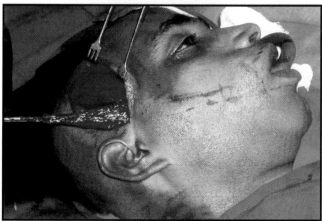

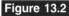

**Figure 13.2**

Temporalis muscle transposition. Four or five muscle slips are transposed to the upper and lower eyelids, upper lip and nasolabial fold, lower lip and commissure. Over correction is essential

enjoyed more popularity than the masseter because of its position, its facility for greater excursion of movement, and its adaptability to the orbit (Breidahl et al, 1996). The technique that is now most widely employed involves two temporal musculofascial strips, which are wound around the zygoma (Fig. 13.3). These musculofascial strips are used to reconstruct upper lip, lower lip and both eyelids. Additional fascial strips can also be anchored to ala of the nose. The technique has several advantages, one of which is that the muscle provides good muscle bulk to compensate lack of fullness on the paralyzed side, in the severely atrophic face. Furthermore, there is direct muscular insertion on the structures to be moved giving greater range of mobilization, and direct muscular insertion enhances chances of myoneurotization.

This procedure is better suited for ocular paralysis, but facial movements are not physiological.

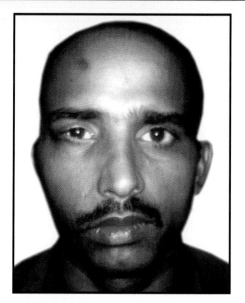

**Figures 13.3 a to c**

Temporalis muscle transposition. (a) Preoperative (b) Temporalis muscle with epicranium attached (c) Postoperative

Because the impulse for muscle movement in temporalis and masseter transfers originates from the trigeminal nerve, facial movement is produced upon chewing, clenching the teeth, and moving the mandible. The basic advantage of masseter and temporalis transfer is the introduction of a large volume of living and dynamic muscle into the face, simplicity of the technique, possibility of myoneurotization, and no loss of other significant function.

2. *Free muscle graft:* In the past, free autogenous muscle graft was also used. The muscle is denervated 14 days before transplantation, full length of the muscle is preserved, and denervated muscle is placed in direct contact with normal, vascularized muscle at the recipient site. The main disadvantages of this procedure are that it is a multistage procedure and it is necessary to intervene on the non-paralyzed side.

   With the present high success rates of microneurovascular muscle transfer, the technique of free muscle grafting has little or no place in the reconstruction of the paralyzed face (McCarthy, 1990).

3. *Free microneurovascular muscle transfer:* The most recent contribution to reanimation of the paralyzed face is the microneurovascular muscle transfer, combined with cross face nerve graft, ipsilateral nerve graft, or split hypoglossal anastomoses. This technique provides new, vascularized muscle to the face that can produce pull in various directions and accomplish more normal facial animation. The advantage over the muscle transfer technique is that the transferred muscle can be reinnervated by a cross face nerve graft, thereby enhancing control of voluntary facial movement. There are certain limitations and at present, it is another alternative in the surgeon's armamentarium of facial reanimation.

   *Choice of donor muscle:* The ideal donor muscle has following criteria.
   1. Excursion should be equal to the normal side of the face.
   2. Reliable vascular and nerve pattern of a size similar to that of the recipient.

3. Removal of the muscle should not leave any functional deficit.
4. Location should be such that two surgical teams should be able to operate simultaneously.

*Gracilis muscle:* (O'Brien et al, 1980). It has a predictable, adequate neurovascular pedicle with adequate bulk. The muscle can be split longitudinally and anterior third of the muscle can be used.

*Pectoralis minor muscle:* (Georgiade, 1992). Its flat shape facilitates insertion in the face. The proximity of the upper chest makes simultaneous two-team dissection difficult.

*Latissimus dorsi muscle and serratus muscle:* They have a predictable neurovascular pedicle and longitudinal intramuscular pattern.

*Rectus abdominis and platysma muscles:* These muscles can also be used.

All of the aforementioned muscles leave minimal or no functional deficit when sacrificed.

*Operative technique:* The operative procedure is usually divided into two stages. The first stage consists in one or more cross-face nerve graft and about 9-12 months later the vascularized muscle is transferred and its neural element is sutured to the distal end of the cross-face nerve graft (Terzis, 1987).

It is important to emphasize that movement of the face after microneurovascular muscle transfer is never normal. Microneurovascular muscle transfer is an alternative surgery for facial paralysis.

The main advantage of the technique is that facial movement is provided and controlled by the contralateral facial nerve, providing for better symmetry and perhaps a more definitive smile. Many disadvantages, however, still exist:
1. There are at least two operative stages with a long surgical time.
2. There are two donor site scars.
3. Usually 2 years elapse before return of facial movement.

4. Complete eyelid closure, forehead movement, oral sphincter, and depressor lip function are almost never restored.
5. The technique is not free of synkinesis and deficit of involuntary emotional expression, common to most other rehabilitative techniques.

### Static Methods of Reconstruction

The static methods of reconstruction of the paralyzed face are the well-known techniques of suspension with fascia lata, tendon, or alloplastic materials. Materials varying from wire, silk, stainless steel and tantalum are also used.

Face lifting and stabilization with dermal flaps have also been used. Reactivation of the facial muscles by neural reconstitution or muscle transposition supersedes any type of rehabilitation by suspension or skin stretching, except perhaps in the elderly or debilitated patient. Static techniques can, however, be complementary to dynamic reconstruction.

*Suspension* (Figs 13.4 and 13.5): Fascia lata is used as a sling for support of orbicularis oris and lower eyelid.

*Mechanical devices:* Various mechanical devices like gold weights (Fig. 13.6), springs (Fig. 13.7) and magnets are used for eyelid closure.

*Selective neurectomy:* Selective sectioning of the intact facial nerve in order to accomplish a more balanced face.

*Selective myectomy:* Various techniques for selective myectomy of the facial muscles to accomplish better balance in repose and during facial expression.

*Surgery for correction to camouflage the deformity:* Various surgical procedures are used to camouflage the deformity. These procedures include excision of nasolabial skin, nasolabial dermofat sling, face-lift, brow-lift, and excision of redundant skin and mucosa.

*Botulinum toxin:* Clostridium botulinum toxin (Botox) is a neurotoxin that temporarily interferes with acetylcholine release from motor nerve endplates, causing skeletal muscle paralysis. The effect lasts for 4-6 months. Botulinum toxin has been useful in the

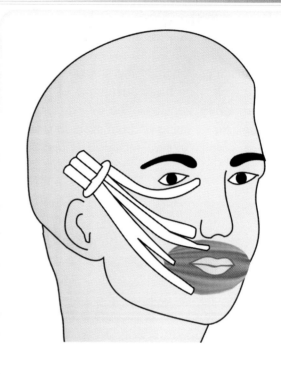

**Figure 13.4**

Fascia lata suspension. The circumoral fascial strip and fascial sling to the lower eyelid is anchored to the temporal fascia by using fascia lata

treatment of facial paralysis by weakening the contralateral side to allow centering of the mouth, more symmetry on smiling, and treatment of hypertrophied platysmal bands.

### SUMMARY

There are many options of treatment, which are available for the patient with a facial nerve paralysis. The treatment goals are directed to the functional and cosmetic deficits that are present and are individualized to suit the patient's needs.

The first goal is to prevent eye complications secondary to corneal exposure. The second goal is to provide functional and cosmetic restoration of the eye, nose, and mouth. These procedures should ideally provide static and dynamic symmetry to the face and allow the patient spontaneous facial animation.

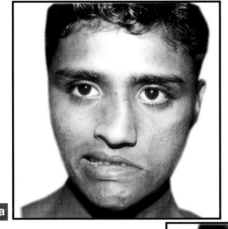
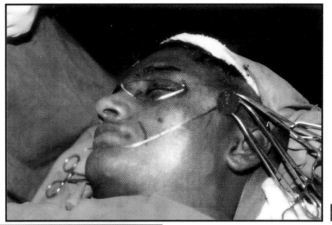
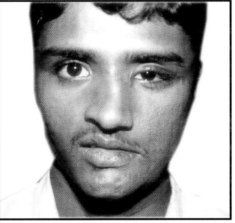

**Figures 13.5 a to c**

Fascia lata suspension. (a) Preoperative (b) Fascia lata to be anchored to orbicularis oris and lower eyelid. (c) Postoperative

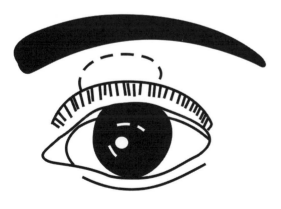
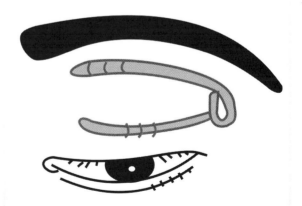

**Figure 13.6**

Weights to aid lid closure. Weight inserted superficial to tarsal plate and deep to orbicularis oculi

**Figure 13.7**

Spring to help eyelid closure. Upper limb sutured to periosteum of supraorbital rim. Lower limb sutured to tarsal plate at eyelid margin

## BIBLIOGRAPHY

1. Breidahl AF, Morrison WA, Donato RR: A modified surgical technique for temporalis transfer. British Journal of Plastic Surgery 1996;49(1):46.
2. Cohen Mimis: Facial reanimation. Mastery of Plastic and Reconstructive Surgery 1994;1045-59.
3. De Castro Correia P, Zani R: Masseter muscle rotation in the treatment of inferior facial paralysis. Plastic and Reconstructive Surgery 1993;52:370.
4. Georgiade Gregory S: Facial paralysis: Principles of treatment. Textbook of Plastic, Maxillofacial and Reconstructive Surgery 1992;581-96.
5. Grabb and Smith: Reconstruction of the paralyzed face. Plastic Surgery 1997;545-57.
6. McCarthy Joseph G: Facial Paralysis. Plastic Surgery 1990;2237-2319.
7. O'Brien BM, Franklin JD, Morrison WA: Cross-facial nerve grafts and microneurovascular free muscle transfer for long established facial palsy. British Journal of Plastic Surgery 1980;33:202.
8. Rayment R, Poole MD, Rushworth G: Cross-facial nerve transplants: why are spontaneous smiles not restored? British Journal of Plastic Surgery 1987;40:592.
9. Sam M Mahaluxmivala: Facial reconstruction. Plastic Surgery—a compendium 1998;59-64.
10. Terzis JK: Reconstructive Micro reconstruction of nerve injuries 1987;170-174.
11. Tolhurst DE, Bos KE: Free revascularized muscle grafts and facial palsy. Plastic and reconstructive surgery 1982;69:760.

❋ ❋ ❋ ❋

# CHAPTER 14
# Facio-hypoglossal Jump Anastomoses for Reanimation of the Paralyzed Face

*JJ Manni*

*"The human face is the most exciting area in the world."*
— *Johan Kaspar Lavator (1741-1801)*

## INTRODUCTION

Preservation of the facial nerve function is a major challenge to the surgeon involved in temporal bone and cerebello-pontine angle surgery. Despite advances in intraoperative facial nerve monitoring, damage to the facial nerve still occurs. A large variety of surgical techniques are available for facial reanimation, with specific indications. Primary end-to-end anastomosis of the facial nerve stumps results in the most optimal functional recovery. To ensure a tensionless facial nerve anastomosis, a nerve graft, or facial nerve rerouting, is often needed. End-to-end anastomosis of the intracranial segment is difficult, because the facial nerve lacks epineurium at this area. Moreover the constant pulsation of the brainstem and the flow of CSF in a deep and narrow wound hamper the technique of anastomosis.

When the proximal stump of the facial nerve is not available for anastomosis, transposition of other cranial nerves to the distal facial nerve stump is a preferred technique. This technique is also indicated when, despite anatomical preservation of the facial nerve, functional recovery does not occur and the muscles of facial expression are still functional.

Transposition of the hypoglossal nerve and end-to-end anastomosis directly to the facial nerve is a popular, effective and reliable technique with constant and satisfying results. However, the complete transection of the hypoglossal nerve inevitably results in homolateral paralysis of the tongue with atrophy, which interferes with mastication, speech and swallowing in particular when the function of muscles of facial expression is less than normal. Moreover, it is emotional for the patient to decide to sacrifice another cranial nerve after having lost the vestibular, acoustic and occasionally the lower cranial nerves or trigeminal nerve as a result of cerebello-pontine angle surgery. Postoperative difficulty in swallowing that was attributed to tongue dysfunction was a complaint of 10 to 12% of patients (Conley and Baker, 1979). Pensak et al (1986) reported that 74% of patients in their series had some functional difficulty while eating, of which 21% were debilitating. Hammerschlag (1989) observed both speech and swallowing problems in 45%. In an effort to reduce the adverse effects Rubin et al (1984) interdigitated the midline tongue musculature using a Z-plasty technique. Other techniques used to reduce the postoperative tongue atrophy were anastomosing of the ansa hypoglossi to the distal stump of the hypoglossal nerve, or longitudinal splitting of the hypoglossal nerve and performing a split XII-VII anastomosis. The results of all these methods were not always encouraging. [Conley and Baker (1979), Kessler et al (1959), Ueda et al (1994), Arai et al (1995)].

In 1991, May et al described a technique wherein the hypoglossal nerve and the facial nerve are anastomosed with the interposition of a free nerve graft, end-to-end to the distal facial nerve stump, and end-to-side to the hypoglossal nerve. The latter is cut in transverse direction for approximately 50% of its diameter. The procedure is indicated in patients with an intact homolateral hypoglossal nerve, an inaccessible central facial nerve stump and a preserved distal facial nerve stump. The activity of the muscles of facial expression should have the potency to be reversible. With this technique the authors observed good facial reanimation and rarely atrophy or impaired movement of the homolateral side of the tongue.

129

## Surgical Technique

The skin incision starts from the insertion of the lobule of the ear slightly curved backward and downward over a distance of approximately 4 cm. The greater auricular nerve is identified and dissected to obtain a graft of about 6 cm length. The facial nerve stump is identified and transected near the styloid foramen together with mobilization of the lateral posterior border of the parotid gland. The hypoglossal nerve is identified just beneath the digastric muscle where it crosses the carotid artery bifurcation and internal jugular vein and it is followed anteriorly to the ansa hypoglossi. The distal end of the graft of the greater auricular nerve is interpositioned end-to-end to the distal stump of the transected facial nerve and the other end sutured end-to-side to the obliquely transected (up to half its diameter) hypoglossal nerve proximal to the ansa hypoglossi (Fig. 14.1). Monofilament 10-0 nylon suture material is used for interrupted epineural tension-free approximation under the operating microscope. Occasionally a Penrose drain is left in the wound. Usually the patient is discharged the second day following the operation. In most of the patients a gold weight is placed on the upper eyelid, after release of an existing tarsorrhaphy.

## Physiotherapy

The patients are advised to follow a physiotherapy program as soon as initial movements in the face appear during tongue movement. The goal of these exercises is to promote facial expression and movements in relation with emotions and expression.

## Personal Experience

The medical records of all patients who underwent hypoglossal facial nerve anastomosis with interposition of a free nerve graft were reviewed. Facial reanimation was assessed in 29 patients who completed 24 months of follow-up. The causes of facial nerve paralysis are summarized in Table 14.1. These 29 patients were placed into 3 groups related to the interval between the onset of facial paralysis and the hypoglossal facial nerve graft anastomosis: Group 1 with an interval from 4 to 12 months, Group 2 with an interval from 12 to 24 months, and Group 3 with an interval of more than 24 months. Group 1 comprised 19 patients (13 females and 6 males) their ages ranged from 11 to 71 years with a mean age of 42.9 years. Group 2 included 6 patients (5 females and 1 male) their ages ranged from 28 to 62 years with a mean age of 41.9 years. Group 3 consisted of 4 patients (1 female and 3 males) their ages ranged from 30 to 62 years with a mean age of 46.7 years. For the evaluation of tongue mobility and appearance, all 29 patients were assessed 6 to 24 months after the operation. Facial nerve function was established using the House-Brackmann (HB) facial nerve grading system (House and Brackman, 1985).

## Results

Improved facial tone and symmetry preceded initial facial movements. In all patients, facial movements appeared at 4 to 18 months, and were usually first observed in the mid-face. We observed that the longer the duration before the operation, the poorer the result. When the duration of paralysis exceeded 2 years, recovery of the muscles of facial expression was poor. Synkinesis was observed in most patients, but no mass movements or gross hypertonia were present. Initial anesthesia due to ablation of the greater auricular nerve appeared insignificant to all patients. Problems with speech, mastication or swallowing were not seen. In a small percentage of patients, slight asymmetry due to reduction in the size of the homolateral tongue were observed. Another small percentage of patients showed no improvement at all.

## Comments

End-to-end anastomosis of the facial nerve stumps either by direct suturing or by interpositioning of a free nerve graft results in the best functional recovery. When the proximal stump is unavailable or when the anatomically preserved facial nerve after cerebello-pontine angle or temporal bone surgery has not regained function and the muscles of facial expression are still viable, transposition of other cranial nerves to rehabilitate these muscles can be considered. The concept of transposition of an alternative motor nerve

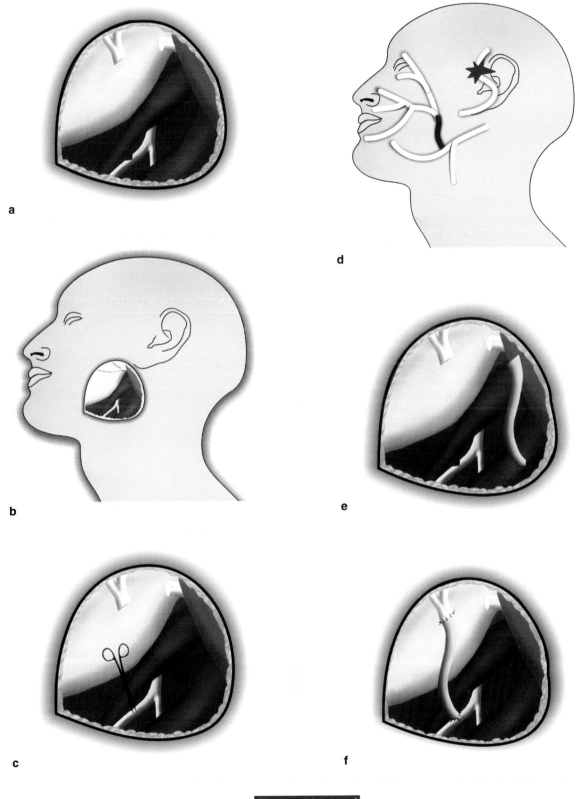

a

b

c

d

e

f

**Figures 14.1 a to f**

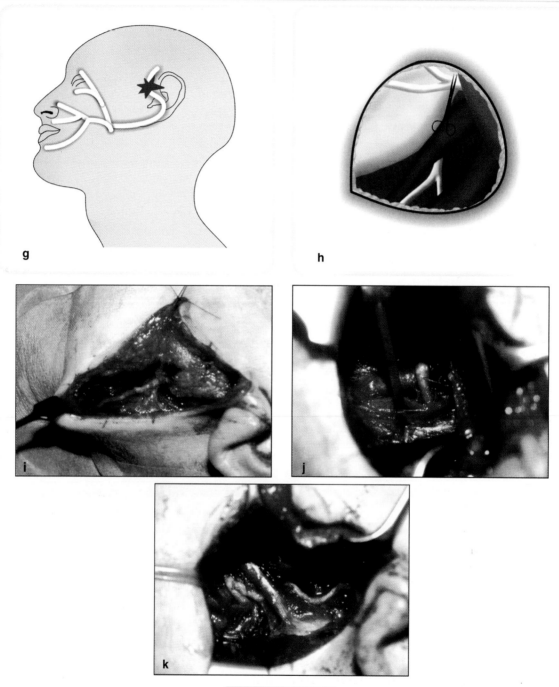

g

h

i

j

k

Figures 14.1 g to k

Figures 14.1 a to k

(a) Facial paralysis not recovered after acoustic neuroma surgery, (b) Overview of regional anatomy, (c) Cutting facial nerve main stem, (d) Transverse cutting of hypoglossal nerve distal from ansa hypoglossi, (e) Result of d, (f) Prepared free graft of greater auricular nerve, (g) End-to-end anastomosis to peripheral facial nerve main stem and side-to-end to hypoglossal nerve, (h) An overview of NVII-NXII jump anastomosis with free nerve graft, (i) Intraoperative view: after skin incision preparation of the free graft of the greater auricular nerve, (j) Intraoperative view: preparation of hypoglossal nerve and ansa hypoglossi crossing the carotid artery, (k) Intraoperative view: free nerve graft anastomosed end-to-side of hypoglossal nerve (arrow) and end-to-end to peripheral facial nerve stem (asterix) guided underneath digastric muscle (see text)

**Table 14.1: Etiology of facial paralysis**

| | |
|---|---|
| Acoustic neuroma | 25 |
| Cerebral infarction | 1 |
| Middle ear malignancy | 1 |
| Supralabyrinthine intracranial cholesteatoma | 1 |
| Plexus chorioideus papilloma | 1 |
| **Total number of patients** | **29** |

**Table 14.2: House-Brackmann facial nerve system**

| Grade | Description | Characteristics |
|---|---|---|
| I | Normal | Facial function in all areas |
| II | Mild dysfunction | Slight weakness noticeable on close inspection; may have very slight synkinesis. At rest: normal symmetry and tone. |
| III | Moderate dysfunction | Gross: obvious but not dis-figuring difference between two sides; noticeable but not severe synkinesis, contracture, and/or hemifacial spasm. At rest: normal |
| IV | Moderately severe dysfunction | Gross: obvious weakness and/or Disfiguring asymmetry and tone. |
| V | Severe dysfunction | Gross: only barely perceptible motion. At rest: asymmetry |
| VI | Total paralysis | No movement |

**Table 14.3: Relation of duration of denervation of muscles of facial expression and expectation of successful rehabilitation**

| Duration of denervation | Functional recovery |
|---|---|
| 1 year | Absolutely certain |
| 1-2 years | Seemingly certain; recommendable |
| 2-3 years | Probable with delay and decrease in functions |
| 3-5 years | Increasingly questionable; patient must be notified |
| 5+ years | Improbable; not to be recommend |

and Woolf, 1992). Taking into account both the duration of facial paralysis and the duration of reneurotization, the decision to perform hypoglossal facial nerve interpositional graft anastomosis is to be taken at latest 1 year after the onset of paralysis in order to obtain the best results. In the presence of an anatomically intact facial nerve and postoperative facial paralysis, nerve function usually showed signs of recovery within 12 months after acoustic neuroma surgery ( Kunihiro et al 1994, Fenton et al, 1999). One may argue that facial nerve regeneration may take up to 18 months before any significant sign of recovery is noted. However, it is questionable if results of recovery will appear as good as with hypoglossal facial nerve graft anastomosis performed at around 12 months after injury, in the absence of clinical and electromyographic signs of recovery. When paralysis lasts more than 2 years, the atrophy of the muscles of facial expression has progressed so far that surgical techniques other than facial nerve reinnervating procedures have to be considered.

Our study confirms the favorable functional results of this technique. Three quarters of our patients achieved HB Grade II and III. The results appear at least as good as the classical, direct hypoglossal-facial

dates back to 1879, when Drobnik anastomosed the spinal accessory nerve to the facial nerve. Other (cranial) nerves used for transposition are: hypoglossal nerve, facial nerve (cross face anastomosis), phrenic nerve, and glossopharyngeal nerve. The major disadvantage of donor nerve techniques is that a functional nerve has to be sacrificed, leaving the patient with functional loss. Results of facial nerve reinnervating surgery are related to the duration of the paralysis, i.e. the functional state of the muscles of facial expression. The functional recovery of denervated muscles is time dependent (Table 14.3) (Stennert, 1979). In addition, the duration of the neurotization also has to be considered. The different steps in neurotization and their duration are summarized in Table 14.4 ( Seckel ,1990, Reynolds

**Table 14.4: Duration of the different stages in neurotization**

| Stages | Duration |
|---|---|
| Sprouting of cranial stump | ± 1 month |
| Passage of nerve suture site | ± 1 month |
| Passage of distal nerve (nerve graft) | ± 1 mm/day |
| Motoric endplate electromyographic activity | ± 2 months |

nerve anastomosis (Conley and Baker, 1979; Hammerschlag, 1999; Brudney et al, 1998; Kunihiro et al, 1994) and preserves tongue function. The best results were acertained in patients undergoing surgery within 12 months after facial nerve injury. This was also shown by others using the classical direct end-to-end anastomosis between both nerves (Conley and Baker, 1979; Stennert 1979; Kunihiro et al, 1994).

In the present study the recovery of the temporal branch of the facial nerve was very poor. This may be related to the observation of Chang and Shen (1984), that the temporal branch contains a relative small number of fibers. However, ineffective function caused by cross innervation of antagonistic muscles in this region and cancelling out each other's activity, a process called *"autoparalysis"* may play a role (Stennert, 1985). We observed less synkinesis with the jump technique in comparison to the classical end-to-end anastomosis. This may be related to the reduced reinnervation. Another explanation could be that, the routinely included physiotherapy may result in more efficient use of the facial musculature.

## BIBLIOGRAPHY

1. Arai H, Sato K, Yanai A: Hemihypoglossal-facial nerve anastomosis in treating unilateral facial palsy after acoustic neurinoma resection. Journal of Neurosurgery 1995;82:51-54.

2. Brudney J, Hammerschlag PE, Cohen HL, Ranshoff J: Electromyographic rehabilitation of facial function and introduction of a facial paralysis grading scale for hypoglossal-facial nerve anastomosis. Laryngoscope 1988;98:405-10.

3. Chang CGS, Shen AL: Hypoglossal facial anatomosis for facial palsy after resection of acoustic neuroma. Surg Neurol 1984;21:282-86.

4. Conley J, Baker D: Hypoglossal-facial nerve anastomosis for reinnervation of the paralysed face. Plastic Reconstructive Surgery 1979;63:63-72.

5. Fenton JE, Chin RYK, Shirazi A et al: Prediction of postoperative facial nerve function in acoustic neuroma surgery. Clinical Otolaryngology 1999;24:483-86.

6. Gidley PW, Gantz BJ, Rubinstein JT: Facial nerve grafts from cerebellopontine angle and beyond. American Journal of Otology 1999;20:781-88.

7. Hammerschlag PE: Facial reanimation with jump interpositional graft hypoglossal facial anastomosis and hypoglossal facial anastomosis: evolution in management of facial paralysis. Laryngoscope 1999;109(suppl 90):1-23.

8. House JW, Brackmann DE: Facial nerve grading system. Otolaryngology and Head and Neck Surgery 1985;93:146-47.

9. Kessler LA, Moldaver J, Pool JL: Hypoglossal-facial anastomosis for treatment of facial paralysis. Neurology 1959;9:118-25.

10. Kunihiro T, Kanzaki J, Yoshihara S, Satoh Y: Analysis of the prognosis and the recovery process of profound facial nerve paralysis secondary to acoustic neuroma resection. Otorhinolaryngology 1994;56:331-33.

11. Kunihiro T, Matsunga T, Kanzaki J: Clinical investigation of hypoglossal-facial nerve anastomosis. European Archives of Otolaryngology 1994;(suppl):3730-35.

12. Manni JJ, Beurskens CHG, Velde van de C, Stokroos RJ; Reanimation of the paralyzed face by indirect hypoglossal-facial nerve anastomosis. American Journal of Surgery 2001;182:268-73.

13. May M, Sobol SM, Mester SJ: Hypoglossal-facial nerve interpositional-jump graft for facial reanimation without tongue atrophy. Otolaryngology and Head and Neck Surgery 1991;104:818-25.

14. Pensak ML, Jackson CG, Glasscock ME, Gulya AJ: Facial reanimation with the twelve-seven anastomosis. Otolaryngology and Head and Neck Surgery 1986;94:305-10

15. Reynolds ML, Woolf CJ: Terminal Schwann cells elaborate extensive processes following denervation of the motor endplate. Journal of Neurocytology 1992;21:50-66.

16. Rubin L, Mishrike YY, Speace G: Reanimation of the hemi-paralytic tongue. Plastic Reconstructive Surgery 1984;84:192-96.

17. Seckel BR: Enhancement of peripheral nerve regeneration. Muscle Nerve 1990;13:785-800.

18. Stennert E: Hypoglossal facial anastomosis: its significance for modern facial surgery II. Combined approach in extratemporal facial nerve reconstruction. Clinical Plastic Surgery 1979;6:471-86

19. Stennert E: The autoparalytic syndrome as cause of permanent loss of function of the frontalis muscle. In: Portmann M (Editor). Facial Nerve. New York: Masson, 1985;291-95.

20. Ueda K, Harri K, Yamada A: Free neuromuscle transplantation for the treatment of facial paralysis using hypoglossal nerve as a recipient motor source. Plastic Reconstructive Surgery 1994;94:808-17.

❋ ❋ ❋ ❋

*C.M. Deshpande, AN Modi*

## INTRODUCTION

The important role of an anesthesiologist in any surgery is not only to give pain relief to the patient; but also to provide an excellent operative field, as hemorrhage is a problem for both the surgeon and the anesthesiologist. In microsurgery of the ear, a near bloodless field is essential. The magnification offered by the operating microscope makes even minimal bleeding appear excessive, thus making surgery very difficult. Since 1917, intentionally reducing arterial blood pressure to hypotensive levels during surgery has been used to provide a good surgical field. When such a deliberate hypotension is combined with the proper positioning of the patient such that the operative site is above the heart level, permitting gravitational venous drainage away from the wound to the dependent portions of the body, the technique has been named *Controlled Hypotension* or *Induced Hypotension*.

## ANESTHETIC AIMS FOR MIDDLE EAR SURGERIES

1. Thorough preoperative preparation which includes:
   a. Anxiolysis
   b. Control and optimization of systemic medical diseases
   c. Treatment of active infection of the surgical site
2. Maintenance of an adequate depth of anesthesia, ventilation and induced hypotensive measures
3. Smooth calm awakening and extubation
4. Prevention of postoperative nausea and vomiting
5. Adequate postoperative analgesia
6. Intraoperative facial nerve monitoring

## Thorough Preoperative Preparation

a. Anxiolysis: To ensure a calm and relaxed patient in the preoperative period.
   This can be achieved by
   • Establishment of good rapport with the patient
   • Benzodiazepines: These cause sedation and anxiolysis
     For example; Oral diazepam 0.2 mg/kg on the night prior to the surgery OR
     Intravenous midazolam 0.03 to 0.07 mg/kg as premedication
   • Antihistaminics: These are beneficial in view of their sedative, anti-tussive and anti-emetic properties.
     For example, Intravenous promethazine 0.5 mg/kg as premedication
   • $\alpha_2$-Adrenergic agonists: For example, Oral clonidine 3-4 mcg/kg as premedication.
   • β-blockers: For example, intravenous metoprolol 0.1 mg/kg as premedication.
b. Optimization of systemic medical diseases like hypertension and uncontrolled diabetes so that hemodynamic instabilities and fluctuations do not lead to troublesome oozing of blood in the surgical field and promote wound healing.
c. Treatment of active infection.

## Induced Hypotension

It is known that a patient who is awake and conscious bleeds less than a patient who is under general anesthesia. However, all patients do not allow surgery under local anesthetic infiltration and any movement of the patient during surgery may hamper success of the operative procedure.

The anesthetist's skill lies in providing conditions that give the surgeon:

i. The best operative field to operate with precision
ii. To permit accurate delineation of lesions without trauma to the surrounding delicate structures
iii. To indirectly help improve viability of grafts and diminish hematoma formation
iv. Reducing overall sepsis and fibrosis

Blood loss during surgery depends on bleeding from the cut vessels. It may be divided into arterial, capillary or venous.

*Arterial bleeding:* It is related to the mean arterial pressure and heart rate. It can be decreased by a reduction in mean arterial pressure or the heart rate.

*Capillary bleeding:* It is dependent upon the local blood flow and can be reduced by local vasoconstriction achieved by infiltration of vasopressors like adrenaline.

*Venous bleeding:* It is related to venous return and venous tone and thus depends on posture. It can be reduced by the use of vasodilators like sodium nitroprusside and nitroglycerine and proper positioning of the patient to promote venous drainage.

*Methods of achieving "Induced Hypotension":* (Simpson et al, 1992).

### Mechanical Methods

*Posture:*

*Effect of posture: a 2.5 centimeter elevation (i.e. a 10-15 degree elevation) of surgical site reduces Blood Pressure by 2 mmHg*

It helps in reducing intraoperative bleeding by:

a. By improving the venous drainage.
b. Producing relative regional ischemia if the operative site is above the level of the heart.
c. Augmenting the effect of agents like sympathetic ganglion blocking drugs.

Thus for surgery in the head and neck region such as the middle ear surgery, a little head elevation is very effective in reducing hemorrhage at the operative site.

### Physiological Methods

1. Effect of intermittent positive pressure ventilation (IPPV) and controlled ventilation: Under normal circumstances venous return to heart occurs during inspiration, when the negative intrathoracic pressure enhances blood flow to the heart. During IPPV, inspiration is associated with positive intrathoracic pressure leading to reduction in venous return which will in turn reduce the mean arterial pressure.

   Thus, IPPV is a useful adjunct to any hypotensive technique as it:

   a. Augments any pharmacological method to decrease the arterial pressure.
   b. Applies positive end expiratory pressure (PEEP) to airways thus limiting venous return and assisting in reduction of arterial blood pressure.

2. Moderate hypocapnea: Carbon dioxide is a vasodilator. Thus reduction in carbon dioxide ($PaCO_2$) to 25 mm of Hg leads to vasoconstriction. Hypocapnea can be achieved by moderate hyperventilation.

### Pharmacological Methods

Mean arterial pressure (MAP) is the most important factor determining the extent of intraoperative bleeding. MAP is directly related to cardiac output (CO) and systemic vascular resistance (SVR).

$$MAP = CO \times SVR$$

Cardiac output is in turn dependent upon myocardial contractility determining stroke volume (SV) and heart rate (HR).

$$CO = SV \times HR$$

Peripheral vasodilatation is controlled by sympathetic activity. Thus, sympathetic blockade leads to vasodilatation leading to decreased venous return and decrease in cardiac output and hence mean arterial pressure.

1. *Local:* Local infiltration using sympathomimetic amines.

Adrenaline is used frequently to induce local vasoconstriction. Concentration should be sufficient to induce vasoconstriction without causing intense or persistent vasospasm. Concentration commonly used is 1:200000 to 1:400000; total dose should not exceed 10 mg/kg.

2. *Systemic*

   a. *Volatile anesthetic agents:* Halogenated inhalational anesthetic agents such as halothane, enflurane, isoflurane and the newer sevoflurane are the most commonly used agents which maintain intraoperative anesthesia and help in reduction of mean arterial blood pressure (Eltringham et al, 1982).

      i. Halothane: It causes moderate degree of peripheral vasodilatation, thus reducing the total peripheral vascular resistance. It also has a direct effect on the myocardium leading to bradycardia and decrease in cardiac output in small concentrations. In higher concentrations, it leads to increased intracranial tension and severe myocardial depression. Thus, it should be avoided in otoneurosurgery.

      ii. Enflurane: The mechanism of action is the same as halothane. The myocardial depression and vagal stimulation is more significant if excessive dose is used. It should be used only in moderate doses.

      iii. Isoflurane: It has minimal effect on myocardium at low inspired concentration. It causes peripheral vasodilatation that can be readily controlled by altering the inspired concentration. It is easily titrable, associated with a rapid recovery and is non-arrhythmogenic, as unlike halothane it does not sensitize the myocardium to endogenous and exogenous catecholamines. It is the agent of choice in otoneurosurgery.

      iv. Sevoflurane: Actions are similar to isoflurane. Because of rapid induction, better hemodynamic profile and rapid recovery it is preferred.

   b. *Muscle relaxants:* Various depolarizing and non-depolarizing agents are used in anesthesia practice. Non-depolarizing muscle relaxants like pancuronium, vecuronium and atracurium are most commonly used in the intraoperative period to achieve muscle relaxation.

      i. Vecuronium: This intermediate acting non-depolarizing muscle relaxant is advantageous in view of its cardiostable properties. It attenuates rise in blood pressure and heart rate, thus maintaining a near normal, in fact, lower pulse rate; aiding our deliberate hypotensive technique.

   c. *Hypotensive agents:*

      i. Alpha adrenergic blockers: These drugs include phentolamine and phenoxybenzamine. The main clinical use of these drugs is for pheochromocytoma and certain hypertensive emergencies.

      ii. Beta adrenergic blockers: These drugs bind selectively to beta-adrenergic receptors and interfere with ability of catecholamines or other sympathomimetics to provoke the beta response. The main advantages of β blockers are the reduction of heart rate and cardiac output by reducing myocardial contractility. Maintenance of a slow heart rate without any additional hypotension controllably reduces bleeding. They can also be used to counteract the tachycardia caused by the ganglion blocking agents or the direct acting vasodilators. Common beta-blockers are propranolol, esmolol, metoprolol, labetelol.

      *Metoprolol*, is a selective beta-1 adrenergic receptor antagonist. It prevents inotropic and chronotropic response while conserving the bronchodilator, vasodilator and metabolic effects of beta-2 receptors intact. Its duration of action is 3-4 hours. It is given in the dose of 0.1 mg/kg intravenously at the time of induction of anesthesia to reduce hypertensive response to intubation and surgical stimulus as well as to reduce intraoperative bleeding. (Benfield et al, 1986).

137

iii. Vasodilators:

a. Sodium nitroprusside: It is an arterial dilator. It allows the rapid reduction in arterial blood pressure and equally rapid restoration to normal value. It is the only drug capable of producing 'Dial a pressure' hypotension over short periods. As a vasodilator it causes an increase in intracranial tension, and so should not be used during neurosurgery before the skull is opened in a patient with increased intracranial tension. A major side effect is cyanide poisoning when used in high doses and over prolonged period. It is used in the dose of 0.3-10 µg/kg/min intravenously to produce controlled hypotension during surgery and anesthesia and for treatment of hypertensive emergencies. An invasive blood pressure monitor is essential while using this drug.

b. Nitroglycerin: It is a venodialator. It produces a steady and less dramatic reduction in arterial blood pressure with greater effect on systolic blood pressure than diastolic blood pressure and therefore, can be used without invasive arterial pressure monitoring. It maintains the blood flow to vital organs and improves coronary blood supply. It is used in the dose of 0.5- 5 µg/kg/min

iv. *Alpha 2 adrenergic agonists:* The perioperative use of α₂- adrenergic agonists is finally coming of age. Since a decade now, clonidine has been registered for clinical use. The clinical responses to α₂-agonists are predictable based on the physiology of the α₂-adrenergic receptors (Takahiko et al, 2000).

**Clonidine** is a selective partial agonist for α₂-adrenoreceptors that decreases sympathetic nervous system output from central nervous system (CNS). It is rapidly and completely absorbed after oral administration and reaches a peak plasma level within 60 to 90 minutes by this route; elimination half-life being between 8-12 hours. Sedation, anxiolysis and anti-sialogogue action are all attractive attributes of clonidine making it a preferred pre-medication agent.

The preanesthetic dose of clonidine has the following advantages:

1. Blunts reflex tachycardia associated with laryngoscopy and intubation.
2. Decreases intraoperative lability of blood pressure thus maintains stable hemodynamics.
3. Reduces plasma catecholamine concentration
4. Dramatically reduces anesthetic requirements of inhaled and injected drugs
5. Prevents postoperative shivering.
6. Preoperative clonidine in doses of 3 to 5 µg /kg is known to decrease postoperative pain and analgesic requirements.

*Use of clonidine in middle ear surgeries is preferred for the following reasons:*

1. Calm sedated patient preoperatively.
2. Smooth induction with attenuated intubation response.
3. Stable hemodynamics in the intra-operative period with mild bradycardia and hypotension enabling maintenance of a clear surgical field.
4. Reduction of anesthetic requirement of nitrous oxide and other anesthetic agents for maintenance of anesthesia.
5. Sedated but rousable and responsive patient in the postoperative period facilitating smooth extubation.
6. Reduction of postoperative nausea and vomiting.
7. Reduction of postoperative analgesic requirement.

*Dose:* 3-5 µg/kg oral tablet in young (18 to 55 years of age) normal patients about 60 minutes prior to surgery give best results.

v. *Propofol:* It is a non-barbiturate induction agent. It has a rapid onset of action which is within one arm-brain circulation time and clinical recovery occurs within 10-15 minutes even after prolonged infusion.

1. Propofol causes fall in systemic vascular resistance leading to hypotension that is greater than one seen with thiopentone.
2. It causes mild bradycardia probably due to central vagal activity.
3. It attenuates pressor response to laryngoscopy and intubation.
4. It is an antiemetic.
5. It depresses pharyngeal and laryngeal reflexes thus laryngospasm and bronchospasm is uncommon with use of propofol.
6. It also reduces the intracranial pressure.

Clinical uses of propofol are as an induction and maintenance agent, hypotensive agent and for its cerebroprotective action.

Dose of propofol in adults is 2-2.5 mg/kg intravenously for induction of anesthesia and 4-12 mg/kg/hr intravenously for maintenance of anesthesia.

*Use of nitrous oxide:* Nitrous oxide is a highly diffusible gas known to enter all body cavities causing them to distend. It diffuses into the middle ear cavity, raising its intracavitatory pressure and distending it. This can have detrimental effects, so ideally, nitrous oxide must be discontinued from the anesthetic mixture about 30 minutes before temporalis fascia graft placement and can be restarted after the same.

## Prevention of Postoperative Nausea and Vomiting

Postoperative nausea and vomiting (PONV) was known to be one of the common sequel of general anesthesia and surgery. However, in this era of modern day-care anesthesia and surgery, the incidence of PONV has decreased considerably owing to:

a. Advances in surgical techniques associated with a reduction in surgical and hence anesthesia time.
b. Use of anesthetic agents with inherent anti-emetic properties.
c. Use of micromotor drills minimizing vestibular stimulation.

Drugs commonly used for prophylactic anti-emesis are:

i. Intravenous metochlorpromide → 0.2 mg/kg before reversal and extubation
ii. Intravenous ondansetron → 0.1 mg/kg before reversal
iii. Intravenous promethazine → 0.5 mg/kg as a premedicant
iv. Intravenous propofol → as a maintenance anesthetic agent as it has significant anti-emetic properties
v. Clonidine.

## Smooth Calm Awakening and Extubation

It is essential to have a sedated, yet arousable patient postoperatively to avoid a stormy recovery.

## Analgesia

Pre-emptive analgesia, i.e. obtaining an adequate state of analgesia without waiting for the patient to complain of pain and then supplementing analgesic medications is the sine-qua-non of modern balanced anesthesia.

## Intraoperative Facial Nerve Monitoring

The probability of iatrogenic injury to the facial nerve during microsurgery of the ear can be reduced by facial nerve monitoring. (Herbert Silverstein, 1991). Anesthesia per se' may interfere with routine facial nerve monitoring and the factors are:

a. *Level of anesthesia:* Light levels of anesthesia have been shown to cause spontaneous muscle contraction artifacts that may be detected by an EMG monitoring system. If the patient awakens, the EMG may get activated. Therefore, it is a must to have an adequate depth of anesthesia around the time that this sort of monitoring is required.
b. *Drugs:* Muscle relaxants may inhibit muscle contractions and electrical activity. Sometimes the effects of these drugs linger and reduce the

sensitivity of the facial nerve to stimulation. Stimulation of peripheral nerves by a stimulator can demonstrate whether the effect of the relaxant is still present; thus using a peripheral nerve stimulator becomes empirical in all cases where facial nerve monitoring is essential.

c. *Electrical interference:* Noise from electrocautery units, video equipment, and other monitoring equipment can cause false muscle contraction artifacts in the EMG monitoring system. Hence as far as possible, the volumes of all monitors inside the operation theater should be kept to a minimum audible tone.

## SUMMARY

Both local anesthesia and general anesthesia have their own applications in otologic surgeries. However, general anesthesia has the advantage of better control over the hemodynamic status and muscle relaxation, which is most important in advanced otologic surgeries. A wider spectrum of surgeries can be done under general anesthesia such as facial nerve decompressions, acoustic neuroma and vestibular nerve sections. Thus, general anesthesia has a definite place in the further advancement of otologic microsurgery.

## BIBLIOGRAPHY

1. Benfield Paul, Clissold Stephen P.—Metoprolol—Drugs 1986;31:376-429.
2. Eltringham RJ. Hypotensive anesthesia for microsurgery of the ear, a comparison between Halothane and Enflurane. Anesthesia 1982;37:1028-32.
3. Herbert Silverstein, Seth Rosenberg. Intraoperative Facial Nerve Monitoring, Otolaryngologic Clinics of North America 1991;24(3):709-14.
4. Simpson P. Perioperative Blood Loss and its Reduction-the role of the anesthetist, British Journal of Anesthesia 1992;69:498-507.
5. Takahiko Kamibayashi,Katsumi Harasawa,Mervyn Maze. Alpha 2 Adrenergic Agonists-:Recent Advances in Anesthesia and Analgesia 2000;21:1-7.

❈ ❈ ❈ ❈

# Index